Easy Hikes

Close to Home

CHICAGO

including
The Collar Counties and Northwest Indiana

TED VILLAIRE

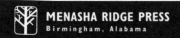

MENASHA RIDGE PRESS
Birmingham, Alabama

This book is meant only as a guide to select trails in the Chicago area and does not guarantee hiker safety in any way—you hike at your own risk. Neither Menasha Ridge Press nor Ted Villaire is liable in any way for property loss or damage, personal injury, or death that result from accessing or hiking the trails described in the following pages. Please be aware that hikers have been injured in the Chicago area. Be especially cautious when walking on or near boulders, steep inclines, and drop-offs, and do not attempt to explore terrain that may be beyond your abilities. To help ensure an uneventful hike, please read carefully the introduction to this book, and perhaps get further safety information and guidance from other sources. Familiarize yourself thoroughly with the areas you intend to visit before venturing out. Ask questions, and prepare for the unforeseen. Familiarize yourself with current weather reports, maps of the area you intend to visit, and any relevant park regulations.

Copyright © 2010 Ted Villaire
All rights reserved
Printed in the United States of America
Published by Menasha Ridge Press
Distributed by Publishers Group West
First edition, first printing

ISBN 978-0-89732-889-0

Cover by Scott McGrew
Cover and interior photos by Ted Villaire
Text design by Annie Long
Maps by Ted Villaire, Steve Jones, and Scott McGrew
Author photo by Michael Roberts

MENASHA RIDGE PRESS
P.O. Box 43673
Birmingham, AL 35243
www.menasharidge.com

Contents

About the Author

Ted Villaire

Ted has hiked, paddled, camped, and bicycled extensively within the western Great Lakes region. As a Chicago resident, he loves getting out of the city to visit nearby scenic hiking destinations. This love of local hiking led him to write *60 Hikes within 60 Miles: Chicago,* from which the hikes in this book are drawn. He is also the author of *Camping Illinois, Best Rail Trails Illinois,* and *Road Biking Illinois.* He edited a weekly Chicago neighborhood newspaper and worked for a number of years as a publications editor for a large Chicago-based non- 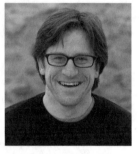 profit. Ted has written freelance articles for a variety of magazines. newspapers, and Web sites. He currently works part-time as writer and editor for the Active Transportation Alliance in Chicago. Ted received a bachelor's degree from Aquinas College in Grand Rapids, Michigan, and a master's degree from DePaul University in Chicago. To contact him and browse photos from each of the destinations in this book, visit **www.tedvillaire.com.**

Introduction

Welcome to *Easy Hikes Close to Home: Chicago*. This book is intended to get you started, or restarted, hiking the best destinations in the Chicago area. The book contains 18 hikes that will enable you to sample the regions's rich assortment of local trails. Because the trails are spread out widely, there's likely one not far from where you live, whether you're in the city, the western suburbs, or northwest Indiana, or near the Illinois–Wisconsin border.

The hikes are organized into three Greater Chicago regions: Cook County and West Chicagoland, North Chicagoland and Wisconsin, and South Chicagoland and Indiana. Numbered map icons on the inside front cover indicate each trailhead and are keyed to the table of contents and narrative text for each trail. On the inside back cover, a map legend defines symbols for parking, restrooms, trail features, and other details.

Each hike description starts with a box that gives you the essential information about the hike: route mileage and configuration, probable hiking time, and brief notes about scenery, sun exposure, park hours, additional maps, restrooms, and other information resources. The description ends with driving directions to the trailhead and public-transit information, if applicable. Those with GPS devices can punch in the trailhead coordinates incorporated into each trail map and let their devices guide the way. Mileage shown for each hike corresponds to the total distance from start to finish; often there are opportunities to shorten or extend a hike with connecting trails.

HIKING ESSENTIALS

Given the gentle landscape in the Chicago region, the best option for hiking footwear is a lightweight low-top hiking shoe. Many hikers also wear regular running shoes, trail runners, sport sandals, or, if they need extra support, hiking boots. I advise against the heavy, stiff hiking boots meant for backpacking with heavy loads over rough terrain. These are simply unnecessary—not to mention expensive. Whatever your footwear, treat your feet well by buying shoes from a specialty store and then breaking them in properly before wearing them on a hike.

Drink water before you hike, carry six ounces of water for every mile you plan to hike, and hydrate after the hike. Pack along a couple of small bottles even for short hikes. You may decide to linger on the trail or take an alternate route and extend your time outdoors. In hot temperatures, bring a greater supply of water and drink more often.

The adage about dressing in layers still holds true. Regulate your temperature by adding and removing layers. Always take at least one more layer than you think you'll need. Many people opt for high-tech, quick-drying fabric over cotton—particularly in hot weather. Hats are hikers' friends, helping keep the sun, rain, and bugs away from your face.

Always plan for unpredictable scenarios by carrying these items, in addition to water:

Trail map	Flashlight
Compass	Rain gear and a sweater or
Basic first-aid supplies, such as	windbreaker, even in warm weather
Band-Aids and moleskin for blisters	Sun protection
Plastic bag for picking up trash	Insect repellent (check periodically for
Pocketknife	ticks, too)
Snacks	Whistle

GENERAL TIPS

The whole point of your outing is to enjoy nature while getting a good dose fresh air and exercise. Here are a few tips to enhance your excursion:

- Be realistic about your fitness level and the mileage you expect to complete. If you're a beginner, start with short hikes and work toward longer ones.

- If your hiking destination is popular, consider avoiding weekends and holidays. Generally, the trails will be less crowded during the week, early in the morning, and during the colder months.

- Double-check to make sure you've packed your map; it'll keep you from getting lost. In the event that you do get lost, retrace your steps back to familiar ground.

- Stay on the existing trail. Unofficial trails cause the trampling of vegetation and erosion.

- Help keep the park clean. Pick up a few pieces of litter and put it in the plastic bag you brought in your daypack.

- When hiking with kids, make sure you match a child's interests and hiking ability with the right trail and the length of time hiking. Take a break every half hour or so.

- Bringing along some easily packed food items will rejuvenate you during the hike. Actual food, such as a sandwich, is always more satisfying than a sports bar. During winter, a thermos filled with hot soup is a hiker's best friend.

- Give wild animals plenty of space. Do not surprise or harass them.

- Be courteous to others you encounter on the trails. Give equestrians the right of way. If cyclists are allowed on the trail, keep a close eye on children, and be mindful of bikes when approaching blind turns.

- Before heading out, check the weather forecast.

TRAIL RECOMMENDATIONS

HIKES WITH BIKING OPPORTUNITIES

HIKES ON LAKES, RIVERS, OR STREAMS

HIKES ON LAKES, RIVERS, OR STREAMS (CONTINUED)

HIKES WITH HISTORIC SITES

SCENIC HIKES

HIKES GOOD FOR BIRD-WATCHING

HIKES GOOD FOR TRAIL RUNNING

HIKES WITH GREAT VIEWS

FLAT OR ALMOST FLAT HIKES

HIKES WITH SOME HILLY SECTIONS

HIKES WITH SOME HILLY SECTIONS (CONTINUED)

HIKES FOR FLOWERS

HIKES ACCESSIBLE BY PUBLIC TRANSIT

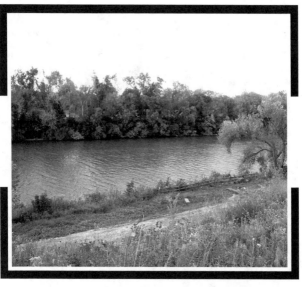

The hike at Lake Katherine runs alongside the Calumet–Sag Channel, a local shipping waterway.

Cook County and West Chicagoland

1 *Deer Grove Loop*

■ OVERVIEW

LENGTH: 5.6 miles	**MAPS:** The Deer Grove Natural Areas Volunteers offer a map at its Web site: deergrove.freehostia.com; U.S. Geological Survey (USGS) topo Lake Zurich, IL
CONFIGURATION: Loop	
SCENERY: Rolling woodland, ravines, streams, and wetland	
EXPOSURE: Shaded	**SPECIAL COMMENTS:** Sections of this trail drain poorly. If you're visiting after a rain, plan on getting some mud on your shoes. During summer, bring mosquito repellent. In winter, Deer Grove is popular with cross-country skiers.
SURFACE: Pavement, dirt, some gravel	
HIKING TIME: 2 hours	
ACCESS: 6:30 a.m.–sunset	
FACILITIES: Restrooms, picnic tables, and shelters	

■ SNAPSHOT

The rolling landscape at Deer Grove is blanketed with thick groves of oak, hickory, and maple. Mixed in with the dense forest are ravines, marshes, ponds, and the occasional stream straddled by picturesque old limestone bridges.

■ UP CLOSE

In 1916, Cook County started acquiring land to create one of the nation's first networks of county forest preserves. The county's first parcel—500 acres that are now part of Deer Grove—was prized for its wooded ravines, winding streams, and marshes and ponds. Over the years, as the size of Deer Grove nearly quadrupled, the preserve was split into two sections. The west section of the preserve, the destination for this hike, encompasses a larger, more heavily forested area, while the east section offers more open space and fewer trails (read about the east section in More Fun).

While Deer Grove claims some of the best hiking in Cook County, the charm of this place has not always been guaranteed. In recent years, sections of the preserve have been plagued by illegal bicycle trails crisscrossing the forest and eroding hillsides.

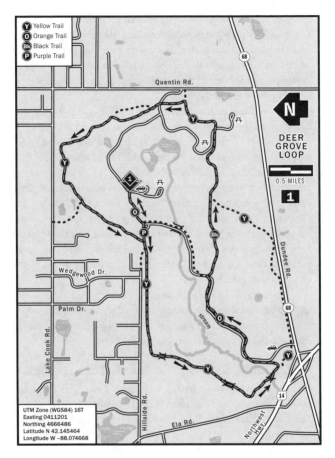

Start the hike on the Orange Trail, which follows an old—sometimes crumbling—narrow paved road. At 0.2 miles, turn right on the Purple Trail, and then quickly turn left on the Yellow Trail. While hiking, keep an eye peeled for buckthorn, an invasive shrub that has been the source of many headaches for the volunteers and county employees who maintain Deer Grove and other natural areas in the region. Since it was imported from Europe in the early

20th century for use on the lawns of lakefront mansions, buckthorn has spread widely throughout Chicagoland. Requiring constant vigilance to keep it under control, buckthorn grows quickly to a height of 20 feet, taking over wooded areas while blocking sunlight for all underlying plants (the oval-shaped leaves are 1 to 2.5 inches long, with fine wavy-toothed edges).

As you approach a large marshy pond on the right, the trail crosses a bridge spanning a small ravine. Turn left on the Orange Trail, which is a former park road. As this paved trail dips and rises, you'll pass a parking area on the right. At 2.6 miles into the hike, turn right on the Black Trail. This wide and fairly flat trail runs through a pleasant oak forest before meeting up again with the Yellow Trail. After turning left on the Yellow Trail, you'll descend a gradual hill, then cross a park road and pass a parking area on the left. On the other side of the park road, the trail accompanies a paved bicycle trail for a bit and crosses a stream. Stay on the Yellow Trail as the paved path cuts right and crosses Quentin Road, providing access to the east section of Deer Grove.

As the trail arcs toward Lake-Cook Road, the woods are dense and the landscape remains flat; if rain has fallen recently, get ready to encounter some mud. To return to the parking lot, turn left on the Purple Trail and then turn left again on the Orange Trail.

■ TO THE TRAILHEAD

From Chicago, follow Interstate 90/94 northwest. After I-94 splits north, follow I-90 for 16 miles to IL 53. Head north for 6.3 miles on IL 53. At North Dundee Road (IL 68), turn left (west) and proceed for 2.9 miles to North Quentin Road. Turn right (north) on North Quentin Road and continue for 0.4 miles until you see the entrance to the preserve on the left. Follow the forest-preserve road for 0.2 miles until you come to the first right. Follow this second unnamed forest-preserve road for 0.6 miles, and then park at the first parking spaces you see on the right, next to the map board.

Public transportation: The Palatine station on the Union Pacific–Northwest Metra Line is less than 2 miles from Deer Grove. From the station, head north on North Smith Street. Two blocks after crossing North Northwest Highway, take the Palatine Trail (paved) left and follow it to the junction of Dundee and Quentin roads. Catch the Black Trail at the northwest corner of this intersection. Follow the Black Trail to the Yellow Trail. Turn right on the Yellow Trail to start the hike.

■ MORE FUN

On the other side of Quentin Road, the east section of Deer Grove contains wooded areas, marshes, and an ample amount of gently rolling open space. There are a couple of miles or so of dirt trails and a 2.5-mile loop of smooth pavement. Park at the picnic area 1 mile east of Quentin Road on Dundee Road or at the Camp Reinberg lot on the east side of Quentin Road, just south of the main entrance for the west side of Deer Grove. You can also walk across Quentin Road on the paved connector trail that accompanies this hike near the main entrance.

2   Crabtree Nature Center Hike

■ OVERVIEW

LENGTH: 2.8 miles	**ACCESS:** 8 a.m.–5 p.m.
CONFIGURATION: 2 connected loops	**FACILITIES:** Exhibit building, restrooms, water
SCENERY: Ponds, marshes, lake, woodland, prairie, and plenty of birdlife	**MAPS:** Available at trailhead; USGS topo Streamwood, IL
EXPOSURE: The prairie is exposed, while the rest of the hike is mostly shaded.	**SPECIAL COMMENTS:** Picnicking is not allowed at Crabtree. The nature center is open March 1–the last Saturday in October, 8 a.m.–5 p.m. daily, and the last Sunday in October–February 28, 8 a.m.–4 p.m. daily. Closed Fridays.
SURFACE: Wood chip, dirt, mowed grass	
HIKING TIME: 1.5 hours	

■ S N A P S H O T

Situated among the rolling hills of far northwest Cook County, Crabtree Nature Center is a place that invites you to linger while admiring wildflowers, spotting waterfowl, and relishing the rapid shifts from prairie to woodland to wetland.

■ U P   C L O S E

The Cook County Forest Preserve District added an attractive parcel to its holdings in the mid-1960s when it bought a country estate and adjoining farmlands and transformed these into the Crabtree Nature Center. Over the years, the county restored the prairie and the scattered plots of woodland that once adorned this 1,100-acre plot. This hike takes place on the western side of the preserve, notable for its varied landscape: prairie, savanna, woodland, ponds, marshes, and a lake are all packed into a small area. Another attraction here is the exhibit building, which offers a collection of handmade displays, as well as a live screech owl, a snapping turtle, plenty of fish, and an enormous bullfrog.

From the parking lot, follow the paved path to the back of the nature center. At the trail board, stay to the right as the trail skirts the edge of Sulky Pond (formerly a sulky track sunken in the ground). The oaks hanging out over the water, the lightly wooded island, and the geese and ducks make this pond an enjoyable spot.

Continue the hike by turning right on the Phantom Prairie Trail. An amusing sign at the beginning of this trail stirs some interest with a warning that this prairie is "not for the meek" because of the harsh winter wind and a lack of shade during the summer. Initially, this trail runs between a woodland on the left and a vast cattail marsh dotted with black willows on the right. Then it winds through a grassy scrubland mixed with goldenrod, staghorn sumac, and cherry trees before reaching a fork. At the fork, head to the right, through the wet prairie toward the stands of quaking aspen and buckthorn trees. Cross an intermittent stream and then emerge in a rolling tallgrass prairie. After brushing against stands of maple and white oak, the trail runs through an area rife with rattlesnake master (round heads dense with little flowers), a member of the

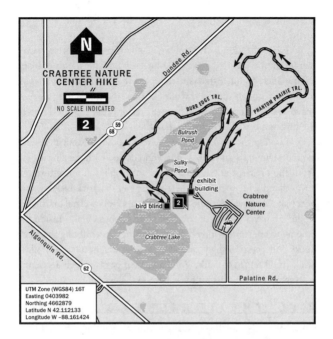

CRABTREE NATURE CENTER HIKE

NO SCALE INDICATED

2

Dundee Rd.

BURR EDGE TRL.

PHANTOM PRAIRIE TRL.

Bulrush Pond

Sulky Pond

exhibit building

Crabtree Nature Center

bird blind   **2**

Algonquin Rd.

Crabtree Lake

Palatine Rd.

UTM Zone (WGS84) 16T
Easting 0403982
Northing 4662879
Latitude N 42.112133
Longitude W –88.161424

parsley family, which at one time was believed to cure rattle-snake bites.

Keep watch at the edges of the prairie for raptors—either perched or soaring. Higher up, you're likely to see (and occasionally hear) a progression of airplanes on the flight path to O'Hare Airport. After passing several small sections of wet prairie, look for honey-locust trees on the right. These trees are unmistakable due to their clusters of thorns—up to eight inches long—growing from the bark. Crossing the boardwalk over the wet, grassy area brings you to the fork that leads back to the Burr Edge Trail.

On the Burr Edge Trail, continue circling the marsh, passing by pasture rose and buckthorn trees as well as walnut and hickory trees wrapped in vines. As you pass under the enormous weeping willows, you'll come upon a pleasant cattail-fringed pond on the left. Along with plenty of waterfowl, the pond is home to muskrats, kingfishers, and, according to park staff, a 40-pound snapping turtle.

From the pond, the trail swings left, passing several silver maples on the way to a grassy area interrupted with stands of black willow and walnut. After you catch a few more fleeting views of the pond through stands of willow shrubs, the trail enters a dense grove of buckthorn followed by a cluster of cattails on one side of the trail and box elder trees on the other side.

Leaving the pond, the trail enters a prairie dominated with big bluestem grass and prairie dock, and dotted with quaking aspen. From the prairie, the trail runs alongside a split-rail fence through a woodland with specimens of maple, pine, shagbark hickory, and burr oak. For now, continue past the Giants Hollow Trail on the left while you pay a visit to the bird blind on Crabtree Lake. Inside the little blind are some handy hand-painted signs identifying the lake's ducks and geese in flight and at rest. Back on the Giants Hollow Trail, you'll return to Sulky Pond and then pass through a savanna with sprawling oaks on your way back to the exhibit building.

■ TO THE TRAILHEAD

Take I-90/I-94 northwest from Chicago. Continue on I-90 for 19 miles after I-94 breaks off. Exit at North Roselle Road and head to the right (north) for 0.9 miles. Turn left (northwest) on IL 62 (Algonquin Road) and drive for 5.3 miles. Turn right (east) on East Palatine Road and go for 0.6 miles. The entrance to Crabtree Nature Center is on the left. From the parking lot, look for signs to the exhibit building.

■ MORE FUN

To the west of Crabtree Nature Center are a couple of hiking opportunities within other Cook County forest preserves. A few miles southwest of Crabtree, and south of I-90, the Poplar Creek Forest Preserve offers a large expanse of woods, prairies, savannas, and wetlands. Follow the trail from the parking lot to the lake and along the top of the dike. After the dike, keep straight ahead until you reach a major trail junction. Hanging a right at the junction takes you on a longer hike through mostly grassland and eventually back to the park road; heading to the left takes you on a shorter hike through woodland and marsh and back to the lake. From Crabtree, take a right on East Palatine Road (IL 62) and turn left on New Sutton Road (IL 59). Follow New Sutton Road until you reach the Shoe Factory Road Prairie parking lot, 0.6 miles south of Shoe Factory Road, on the right.

Northwest of Crabtree, trails also can be found among the lakes, grasslands, woods, and marshes at the Spring Creek Valley Forest Preserve. In the southern section of the preserve, 2.4 miles of established trails are accessible from the Beverly Lake parking area. Starting from the shore of Beverly Lake, the loop begins after a half mile of hiking. Follow the entire loop or shorten the hike via connector trails. Several hiking and bridle trails are accessible from the dog-training area to the west along Higgins Road. Bring a GPS device, however, because these trails can be confusing. To reach Beverly Lake, follow the directions to Poplar Creek Forest Preserve. As you're heading south on New Sutton Road, turn right on West Higgins Road (IL 72). The parking area is 2.1 miles ahead on the right.

3 Fullersburg Woods Forest Preserve Loop

■ OVERVIEW

LENGTH: 3.25 miles	**FACILITIES:** Visitor center, restrooms, water, benches, and numerous log picnic shelters alongside the trail
CONFIGURATION: Loop that includes a couple of short loops	
SCENERY: Salt Creek, woodland, marshes, islands, footbridges, and a mill that is now a museum	**MAPS:** Available outside the visitor center; USGS topo Hinsdale, IL
EXPOSURE: More exposed than shaded	**SPECIAL COMMENTS:** The visitor center is open 9 a.m.–5 p.m., except major holidays, and can be reached at (630) 850-8110. The mill is open mid-April–mid-November, Tuesday–Sunday, 10 a.m.– 4:30 p.m. Admission to the mill is $3.50 for adults. Call (630) 655-2090 or visit www.dupage forest.com for more information.
SURFACE: Crushed gravel	
HIKING TIME: 2 hours, including a visit to the Graue Mill	
ACCESS: 1 hour after sunrise–1 hour after sunset	

■ SNAPSHOT

You may be surprised to find this much natural beauty just 20 miles from the Loop. Nearly all of this hike accompanies Salt Creek as it meanders next to a bluff and winds around a couple of islands on its way to the historic water mill at the south tip of the park.

■ UP CLOSE

Nestled against the communities of Hinsdale, La Grange, and Oak Brook, the 222 acres of Fullersburg Woods Forest Preserve have been a popular spot since opening to the public in 1920. While visitors have always been drawn to the creek and its environs, more recently the historic mill and visitor center have served as added attractions. When you pick up a map at the door of the visitor center, be sure to duck inside to see the 13,000-year-old woolly-mammoth skeleton. The skeleton was uncovered in 1977 at Blackwell Forest Preserve, about 15 miles west of Fullersburg. The accompanying signs describe how researchers determined

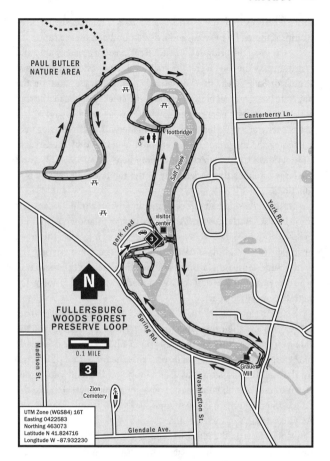

PAUL BUTLER
NATURE AREA

footbridge

Canterberry Ln.

Salt Creek

York Rd.

visitor
center

park road

N

**FULLERSBURG
WOODS FOREST
PRESERVE LOOP**

0.1 MILE

3

Spring Rd.

Graue
Mill

Madison St.

Zion
Cemetery

Washington St.

UTM Zone (WGS84) 16T
Easting 0422583
Northing 463073
Latitude N 41.824716
Longitude W −87.932230

Glendale Ave.

the animal's age at death and gender and why researchers disagree about whether the mammoth was killed by humans. Kids will also enjoy a few mounted animal specimens, interactive displays, and the spotting scopes pointed toward Salt Creek.

To start the hike, look for the crushed-gravel trail on the north side of the visitor center. After you pass a wide point in the creek, continue straight ahead over the bridge and turn left. During the short stroll around the island, you'll pass a picnic shelter, tree stumps sculpted by beavers, and a dried pond bed on the right.

Crossing the bridge again, turn right, passing a water pump and restrooms on the left. Here, the trail meanders beside an attractive stretch of Salt Creek: trees hang lazily over the water, and, on the opposite bank, a small bluff rises above the creek. Just ahead, the trail passes an impressive stone picnic shelter with benches and a fireplace. Many of the Fullersburg picnic shelters, as well as the log visitor center and the Graue Mill, were built or restored by the Civilian Conservation Corps, which had a camp here in the 1930s. Beyond the large boulders on the left, stay to the right at the next five trail junctions.

After crossing Salt Creek again, you'll pass a trail heading left into the Paul Butler Nature Area. If you wish to add an extra mile or so to your hike, take this narrow footpath as it follows the creek upstream to a small dam. When you reach the pond beyond the dam, I suggest turning around and heading back to the main trail (the remainder of this trail can be flooded in spots and is noisy due to traffic on 31st Street).

Continuing on the main trail, the path curves left, away from Salt Creek, and then rises up a small hill. As the path returns to the side of the creek, look for the trail you just hiked on the other side of the creek. On the left, you'll soon pass the other end of the trail for the Paul Butler Nature Area. Not long after the landscape drops down to creek level, you'll pass over a couple of small streams; the first is intermittent, and the second looks as if it runs year-round. As you pass the island you hiked earlier, you'll start to see backyards of houses on the left. At 1.9 miles into the hike, a picturesque log bridge leads over Salt Creek to the visitor center.

After the bridge, the path runs straight south as the stream slowly curves to the right. When you meet back up with the creek, the water grows wider until you reach the dam, which is flanked by the brick Graue Mill and its giant waterwheel. For anyone with an interest in local history and water mills, the Graue Mill is well worth a visit. Cross York Road on the footpath and head over to the front door of the mill, which faces the former Graue House.

The owner of the mill, Frederick Graue, once lived here with his family.

For a small admission fee, you can hear a 20-minute presentation in which a white-aproned miller explains the 15,000-year-old practice of grinding grain and how it was done here. After Frederick Graue built the mill in 1852, three generations of his family operated the mill until 1912, and it continued as a working mill until 1929. At the end of the presentation, the miller grinds a half-bucket of cornmeal using the mill's original millstones, which are made from a type of quartz—known as buhrstone—imported from France. While the millstones are now powered by electricity, sets of giant wooden gears in the basement are set up as they would have been when the waterwheel powered the millstones.

In the basement, you'll learn that the mill was also a stop on the Underground Railroad. Along with other local stops in Plainfield, Aurora, Sugar Grove, Joliet, and Hinsdale, the Graue Mill was a part of the clandestine network of places where escaped slaves could rest and be fed on their way to Chicago, from which they could travel across the Great Lakes to Canada. On the second and third floors of the mill is a collection of artifacts from the period of 1850 to 1890, including room settings, farm implements, and a re-created general store.

From the mill, the path runs back to the visitor center between the dam's backwater and Spring Road. Along the way, you'll pass a sign explaining that Salt Creek got its name when a farmer's wagon was stuck in the creek while hauling a barrel of salt. He left the wagon overnight and returned the next morning to find the salt had dissolved. Farther ahead, follow the trail branching to the right. Then take the short bridge to the right for a short loop around this little piece of land—sometimes an island—that sticks out into the water. Crossing back over the bridge, continue to the right until you see the parking lot on the left.

■ TO THE TRAILHEAD

From Chicago, take I-290 west to I-88. Follow I-88 for 3.5 miles until you reach IL 83 (Kingery Highway). Follow IL 83 south for

0.8 miles. Turn left (east) on 31st Street and travel 0.5 miles until you turn right (south) on Spring Road. Turn left 0.6 miles ahead at the sign for Fullersburg Park. The visitor center is at the north end of the parking lot.

■ MORE FUN

If you'd like to see more of Salt Creek, head to Bemis Woods Forest Preserve, 1 mile directly east of Fullersburg Forest Preserve. Bemis Woods offers several miles of multipurpose trails and the western end of the Salt Creek bicycle path. This paved path runs for 6.6 miles east, ending at the doorstep of the world-renowned Brookfield Zoo. To reach Bemis Woods, turn left (southeast) on Spring Road as you're leaving Fullersburg Park. After passing the Graue Mill, turn left (south) on York Road. Turn left (east) on Ogden Avenue and proceed for 1.2 miles. The driveway for Bemis Woods is on the left. The bicycle trail starts on the right, just before the sledding hill.

4   *Morton Arboretum East Hike*

■ OVERVIEW

LENGTH: 5 miles	**MAPS:** Available from attendant at the gate; USGS topo Wheaton, IL
CONFIGURATION: 2 connected loops	
SCENERY: Rolling hills, dense woods, oak savannas, and prairie	**SPECIAL COMMENTS:** Runners are asked to use the roads rather than the trails. Cross-country skiing is not allowed. For information about guided tours on an open-air tram, inquire at the visitor center.
EXPOSURE: Mostly covered	
SURFACE: Wood chips, dirt	
HIKING TIME: 2.5 hours	At the visitor center, learn about scores of classes the arboretum offers. For more information call the main office at (630) 968–0074 or visit the arboretum's Web site at www.morton arb.org.
ACCESS: April–October, 7 a.m.–7 p.m.; November–March, 7 a.m.–5 p.m. Cost is $9 for adults, $8 for seniors, $6 for kids.	
FACILITIES: Restrooms, benches, picnic tables, water, visitor center, cafe, arboretum shop, public phone	

■ SNAPSHOT

Want to check out trees from places such as Korea or Appalachia? Or maybe you'd like to see a sampling of the 43 types of oak trees and 60 types of maple trees that grow here. Tree lovers could be busy for weeks exploring the hundreds of types of trees grouped according to geographical origin, species, and habitat. But trees are just part of the appeal of this place. The gently rolling terrain offers plenty of scenic beauty in the way of native woodlands, savannas, streams, marshes, and ponds.

■ UP CLOSE

Occupying 1,700 acres of rolling wooded terrain and bisected by the East Branch of the DuPage River, the Morton Arboretum will captivate anyone with even a slight interest in woody vegetation. Joy Morton, founder of the Morton Salt Company, established the arboretum on his country estate in 1922. Morton's arboreal interests were passed down to him from his father, Julius Sterling Morton, who served as Secretary of Agriculture under President Grover Cleveland and who founded Arbor Day (typically the last Friday in April, but the date varies from state to state).

Joy Morton's plan for the arboretum was to gather trees and shrubs from around the world that could farr well in the Northern Illinois climate. In the first year, the arboretum planted 138,000 trees; now there are some 3,400 varieties of plants and trees, many of them organized according to botanical groups (such as elm, maple, oak, willow, and spruce trees) and geographical origins (such as Japan, China, Appalachia, and Northern Illinois). Mixed in with this extraordinary collection of trees and shrubs are a variety of gardens highlighting herbs, native plants, and hedges.

Most of this hike follows the outer edge of what's called the Main Trail, which is a series of four connected loops numbered from west to east. Facing the Big Rock Visitor Station, look for Main Trail Loop 3 to the left, heading west across the park road from the shelter. Passing a picnic spot, the trail enters rolling open terrain, with the occasional bluebird house attached to a post. At

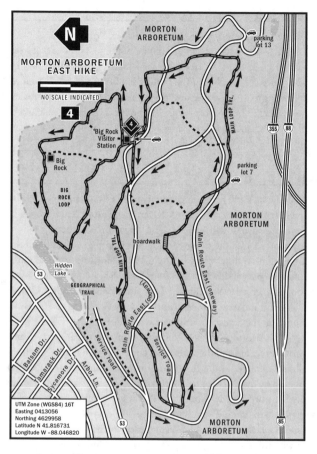

0.2 miles, you'll see a connector trail that runs left into a bulb meadow and through collections of beech and maple trees. Continuing on the Main Trail, you'll cross a park road and soon enter flat, dense woodland with the occasional stand of spruce. At a half mile into the hike, where the woodland gives way to shrubby trees and more open space, you'll cross a wooden footbridge spanning a small ravine.

Up ahead, as the trail crosses the park road, a sign indicates that the plants of Appalachia have been planted in this area. After passing another connector trail on the left, the path runs next to one striking Appalachian specimen—the northern catalpa tree, identified by its long, thin, beanlike fruit and large, showy flowers that bloom in the spring. Gradually descending a gentle hill, the trail is accompanied by a small stream on the right. At 1 mile into the hike, a sign on the right announces the beginning of the Geographical Trail, a short loop showcasing the trees of China and Japan. Continuing on the Main Trail, you'll pass a collection of maples and then cross a service road that brings you into a collection of azaleas, rhododendrons, and other types of ornamental shrubs. The trail quickly rises to a small stone platform with a couple of benches. Behind the bench on the right is an Eastern redbud tree, which produces masses of pink flowers in early spring; behind the other bench is another flowering tree, the wild black cherry.

From the benches, take the trail to the left past plantings of locust, honeysuckle, and viburnum trees. In the open space on the right are a small pond and the park road at the far edge of a clearing. As the trail enters an area with plants from Korea, look for trees common in Asia—such as mock orange and koyama spruce—that are marked on the side of the trail. After passing a grouping of large hedges, the Crowley Marsh appears on the right, soon followed by a connector trail on the left. Cross the park road and you'll enter an area planted with trees from the buckeye family. As the trail curls around Burr Reed Marsh, you'll mount a short boardwalk and viewing platform that affords an ideal spot from which to look for birds during migratory months.

Passing another small pond and another connector trail, keep straight ahead as you enter a savanna and woodland area containing 43 types of oaks from around the world. Among these you'll find six main types of oaks growing in the Chicago region: white, swamp white, bur, black, red, and Northern pin. After leaving the oaks, cross the park road and then pass by parking lot 7. Keep straight ahead at the next junction, which appears alongside a winding creek bed.

Here the trail straightens and starts to rise gradually as it cuts through a fairly dense woodland. The stands of shrubs and abundant deadfall seem to draw in the critters. On one of my visits to this corner of the arboretum a couple of days after a snowfall, the hiking trail was crisscrossed with countless animal trails, some apparently used by more than one type of animal. Raccoons, mice, squirrels, rabbits, chipmunks, and deer all left behind their imprints. Along this section of the trail in winter, I've also seen large patches of ground where deer had kicked up oak leaves from underneath the snow—presumably to find a stray acorn or two.

Stay to the left at the sign for Parking Lot 13, and then cross the park road again. After crossing over a bridge, the trail slopes down lazily while accompanying a dry streambed. Crossing the road again, the landscape regains its rolling quality. Here, the trail skirts a wooded hillside above a picturesque ravine sprinkled with fallen trees. Soon, on the left, you'll pass a trail that leads—if you care to take it—to a plot of spruce trees. Continuing straight ahead brings you back to the Big Rock Visitor Station.

For a quick introduction to the types of environments within this section of the arboretum, follow the short paved path bordering the backside of the visitor station and peruse the informational signs along the way.

Find the beginning of the Big Rock section of the hike next to the shelter. Fifty yards ahead, turn right at two closely spaced trail junctions. After the second junction, the trail proceeds alongside a small stream on the right that has carved a shallow ravine. Growing in these low spots amid the deadfall are trees tolerant of moist soil, such as red oak, basswood, and green ash. As the trail swings left and slowly starts to rise, you'll see trees that require drier ground, such as white oak, maple, and ironwood. Off to the right, the landscape drops down toward power lines and a marshy area. While the trail curves, dips, and rises through fairly dense woodland, keep an eye out for a few enormous white oaks. (Growing to 100 feet, the white oak—the Illinois state tree—has wide-spreading branches, leaves with rounded lobes, and ashen-gray bark that is plated and scaly.) After passing a junction on the right, the trail gradually descends toward a rock the size of a small car.

Weighing in at 12 to 14 tons, the Big Rock hitched a ride on a glacier many thousands of years ago from either northern Michigan or Canada. Geologists point to particular surface scratches on the rock and its position on the ground as possible evidence that farmers moved it out of the adjoining field about 100 years ago. Up until the 1980s, the clearing west of the rock operated as a hay field.

Passing a trail junction on the left, proceed straight ahead into the former hay field. Now a restored prairie, this big open space is bordered by oaks and a few stands of birches. After a quarter-mile hike through the prairie, the trail crosses a two-wheel track, then enters a savanna that is often alive with avian activity: look for woodpeckers, flickers, juncos, and cedar waxwings in the winter and a host of migrating species such as warblers, vireos, and scarlet tanagers in the spring and fall. Local bird-watchers say that the arboretum's variety of plants and berries makes it one of the better birding spots in the area. After crossing a small bridge, the trail gradually turns left, then starts to rise into dense woods. Stay right at the next two trail junctions on your way back to the Big Rock Visitor Station.

■ TO THE TRAILHEAD

From Chicago, take I-290 west to I-88. Follow I-88 for 10.5 miles until you reach IL 53. The entrance to Morton Arboretum is just a quarter mile north on IL 53, on the right. After paying at the gate and receiving a map, follow Main Route East Side for 2.5 miles until you reach the Big Rock Visitor Station, which will appear on the right side of the road.

Public transportation: The arboretum is 1.5 miles away from the Lisle station on the BNSF Railway Metra line. From the north side of the station, head west on Burlington Avenue. Turn right (north) on Lincoln Avenue (IL 53). Use care while walking or riding along Lincoln Avenue—it's a busy road. The entrance to the arboretum is on the right after you pass under I-88.

■ O V E R V I E W

LENGTH: 1.35 miles	**SPECIAL COMMENTS:** During the past couple of decades, Jackson Park has become much safer. Crimes such as muggings are rare. Still, while walking in any urban area, be mindful of your surroundings. When walking in unfamiliar urban terrain, it's never a bad idea to walk with a companion. The Jackson Park Advisory Council offers a great Web site with extensive information about the park and the World's Columbian Exposition: www.hyde park.org/parks/jpac.html.
CONFIGURATION: Loop	
SCENERY: Lagoon, islands, Japanese garden, meadow, open parkland	
EXPOSURE: Half shaded, half exposed	
SURFACE: Pavement, dirt	
HIKING TIME: 30–45 minutes	
FACILITIES: Drinking fountain, restroom	
MAPS: USGS topo Jackson Park, IL	

■ S N A P S H O T

At the heart of Jackson Park is a wooded island containing a serene Japanese garden and placid lagoons lined with cattails. Much of this quiet refuge is a remnant of one of the most important events in Chicago history: the World's Columbian Exposition of 1893.

■ U P   C L O S E

In preparation for Chicago's 1893 World's Columbian Exposition, a team of the nation's most significant architects and sculptors came to the grounds of Jackson Park to create the "White City," made largely of plaster buildings designed in a classical style. The city included sculptures, fountains, and some 200 buildings exhibiting art, machinery, animals, plants, food, and other items. The exposition was an absolute success: more than 27 million people attended this event, held to celebrate 400 years of post-Columbus civilization. After the exposition, the city converted the ground's 700 acres—from East 56th Street south to East 67th Street, and from the shoreline west to South Stony Island Drive—back to a city park.

While the exhibition was not meant to be permanent, one notable exception was the sprawling Palace of Fine Art, which was

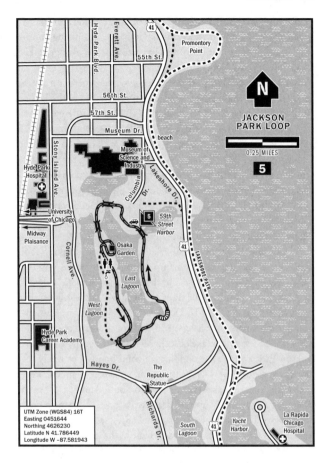

UTM Zone (WGS84) 16T
Easting 0451644
Northing 4626230
Latitude N 41.786449
Longitude W –87.581943

eventually converted into the Museum of Science and Industry. Another attraction left over from the exposition is a lovely Japanese garden, one of the first stops on this ramble through Jackson Park.

The hike starts on the west side of the parking lot, on the bridge overlooking a pool lapping at the back steps of the museum. This bridge is named after Clarence Darrow, a famous Chicago defense lawyer who was one of the many speakers at the 1893

Exposition. On the other side of the bridge, looking south, is the East Lagoon, along with a wooded island and a sprinkling of other tiny islands. After crossing the Clarence Darrow Bridge, take a quick left to cross North Bridge.

Over the bridge, pass through the wooden gates on the left to enter a storybook Japanese garden on the shore of the lagoon. Built for the Columbian Exposition in 1893, the garden was virtually abandoned after World War II, then was rebuilt in 1981. In 1993, the garden was renamed the Osaka Garden in honor of Chicago's sister city in Japan. While walking along the 0.15-mile winding gravel path, lined with red granite blocks taken from Chicago's old streetcar tracks, you'll enjoy a pleasant waterfall, stone lanterns, and a little bridge arching over a rock-lined lily pad pond. The teahouse, added to the garden in 1981, is one of many places where you can have a seat and enjoy the view.

Continuing south on the island, you'll pass drinking fountains and a portable restroom just beyond the garden entrance. Take either route at the fork: both trails lead through a densely wooded area and offer spur trails to the shore of the lagoon. Formally known as the Paul H. Douglas Nature Sanctuary, this small island is a hot spot for birders: 250 bird species have been sighted here, while 55 species make nests here. One bird species dwelling in Jackson Park and the surrounding neighborhoods, but rarely seen elsewhere around Chicago, is the monk parakeet—a green, loudly chattering, medium-sized bird native to South America. Since the parakeets mysteriously appeared a few decades back, their origin has remained a matter of speculation: some say they were pets set free; others say they escaped from a crate at the airport.

At the southern tip of the island, cross the bridge and then cut left along the shoreline. First, however, you may want to take a short detour straight ahead to Hayes Drive and then left to South Richardson Drive to visit an impressive shining bronze statue called *The Republic,* a replica of the much larger statue that was built for the Columbian Exposition.

Continuing along the shore of the lagoon, you'll pass groves of weeping willows and a lagoon featuring prairie plants. After

0.2 miles hiking along the shore of the lagoon and past the soccer fields on the right, follow the boardwalk that starts at the limestone fishing platform. Stay left through the small parking lot to the beginning of the trail through Bobolink Meadow.

Largely ignored by human visitors, this meadow is alive with animals and plants: rabbits scurry across the trail and songbirds serenade each other while perched on big bluestem, Indian grass, goldenrod, and other prairie plants. On your left, several side trails lead toward the trees drooping lazily over the water. Prior to the Columbian Exposition, this was a swampy marshland. Later it was used for athletic fields, and, surprisingly, from 1956 to 1971, it hosted an Army missile base. Since 1982, this plot has served as a nature preserve. Stay left as you pass through the gate, and head toward the bridge overlooking 100 or so boats moored in 59th Street Harbor. Continue along the shore of the lagoon, straight ahead to the parking lot.

■ TO THE TRAILHEAD

Exit Lakeshore Drive at the Science Drive exit (just south of the 57th Street exit). Stay left as you enter the parking lot, next to the lagoon at the backside of the Museum of Science and Industry.

Public transportation: Take the South Shore Line to the 59th Street station. On East 59th Street, head east (toward the lake), crossing South Stony Island Avenue and South Cornell Avenue, for 0.3 miles to the Clarence Darrow Bridge.

■ MORE FUN

While visiting Jackson Park, consider taking a short walk to Promontory Point, perhaps the best slice of open parkland in the city. From the parking lot where the hike starts, head toward the lake on the paved path that runs on the north side of the harbor. After passing a lawn-bowling green on the left, the path enters a tunnel under Lakeshore Drive. Emerging from the tunnel, turn left and continue past the beach, arriving at Promontory Point 0.4 miles north of the tunnel. Known simply as "The Point," the park occupies a small piece of land jutting into the lake and offers plenty of benches and big rocks from which to enjoy a great view of the downtown skyline.

Walking west of the parking lot where this hike starts, you'll encounter the southern edge of the University of Chicago campus and the Midway Plaisance, a mile-long strip of green space running east–west. During the Columbian Exposition, the Midway Plaisance hosted amusement rides and a collection of re-created villages from around the world; now, it's open parkland with statuary and an ice rink operating in the winter. Starting at the east end of the Plaisance—closest to Jackson Park—you'll pass the large round Perennial Flower Garden, a statue of St. Wenceslas, the Rockefeller Memorial Chapel (with dozens of outdoor statues of religious figures), another garden, and several university residence halls.

Architecture fans will enjoy the English Gothic style that characterizes many of the University of Chicago's buildings. To see more of the campus, turn right on South Woodlawn Avenue, just east of the Rockefeller Chapel. One block ahead, turn left on East 58th Street toward the center of campus. At the northeast corner of Woodlawn and 58th, don't miss Frank Lloyd Wright's Robie House—considered the most complete expression of the architect's Prairie School style. Call (773) 834-1847 for tours.

For information about the Museum of Science and Industry's hours and admission prices, call (773) 684-1414 or visit **www.msi chicago.org.**

OVERVIEW

LENGTH: 3.2 miles	exhibits, and an ice-skating rink in winter
CONFIGURATION: Combo	
SCENERY: Lake, canal, woodland, specialty gardens, man-made waterfalls	**MAPS:** Available from the learning center; USGS topo Palos Park, IL
EXPOSURE: Mostly shaded	**SPECIAL COMMENTS:** Dogs must be leashed and picked up after. The environmental learning center is open Monday–Friday, 8:30 a.m.–5 p.m., and weekends, 8:30 a.m.–4 p.m. Closed Sundays during winter months. Call (708) 361-1873 for more information.
SURFACE: Wood chips, dirt, gravel	
HIKING TIME: 1.5 hours	
ACCESS: Sunrise–10 p.m.	
FACILITIES: Benches, restrooms, an environmental learning center with	

SNAPSHOT

As an urban nature walk, this is one of the best in the area. Nestled alongside the Calumet–Sag Channel, the 136-acre Lake Katherine Preserve features an attractive lake, an arboretum, a waterfall garden, an herb and conifer garden, and expansive views from atop a ridge in the eastern section of the preserve.

UP CLOSE

In the 1980s, this patch of land was an eyesore. People had left mounds of debris and junk amid piles of boulders and overgrown bushes. Then the city of Palos Heights decided to transform it into parkland. The result is a charming urban park, half of which is carefully landscaped and the other half fairly wild. In 1992, then–First Lady Barbara Bush presented the preserve with a National Landscape Award, sponsored by the American Association of Nurserymen.

Much of this hike runs alongside the Calumet–Sag Channel, a 16-mile waterway between the Little Calumet River and the Sanitary and Ship Canal. Slow-moving barges frequently use this

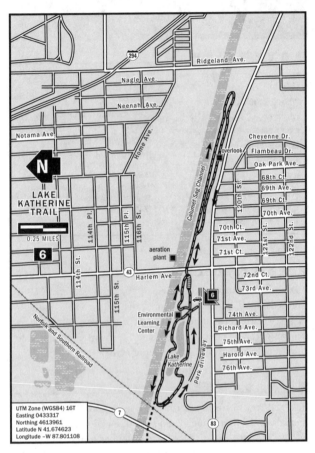

channel to transport cargo such as fuel oils, coke, and gasoline between the Mississippi River and Calumet Harbor, the largest harbor on the Great Lakes. The digging of the channel started in 1911 for the purpose of creating a feeder channel for the Illinois and Michigan Canal. It also brought polluted water away from Lake Michigan, keeping Chicago's drinking water safe and clean. In the following years, after the channel was widened and dredged, it proved to be an important shipping route.

From the parking lot, head toward the buildings on the edge of the lake. The first building on the right is the E. G. Simpson Clubhouse—a remnant of a former gun club that is now used for banquets. After passing the small pier and the environmental learning center, which caters largely to school groups, you'll see a small herb garden with dozens of plants growing in raised beds. If you've ever wondered what curry, horseradish, lavender, oregano, or basil plants look like, here's your chance to find out. Next is a bird-and-butterfly garden hosting a variety of shrubs, flowers, grasses, and vines meant to attract the winged creatures.

Continuing on the wood-chip trail brings you past a cluster of conifer trees and a bench overlooking the canal. Farther along is an observation platform at the edge of the lake. At the sign for the children's forest, continue straight ahead and then, before the bridge, take the trail on the left, leading you into an area dense with cottonwood and shrubs. If you continue ahead, you can hike for another third of a mile under two bridges—one that serves the Norfolk and Southern Railroad and one that serves IL 7. The children's forest on the left had its beginnings on Arbor Day in 1990, when some 500 children and their families planted trees and bushes on this several-acre plot.

As you walk parallel to the train tracks up on the embankment, stay left and cross a wooden bridge over an intermittent stream. Keep straight ahead through the children's forest until you're back at the wood-chip trail near an arch from the front doorway of a former Palos Heights elementary school. Continuing around Lake Katherine to the right, the shoreline opens up, providing a view of the cattails, sedge grasses, and lily pads out in the water.

While conifers and cottonwood grow fairly thickly on the north side of the lake, the south side hosts about 70 different tree species, many of them identified with plaques. Along with more than a dozen crab apple trees, there are silver maple, burr oak, gingko, locust, green ash, American filbert, and swamp white oak. As the trail winds around the lake, multiple benches are situated on the little pieces of land jutting into the lake. On the wooded island across from one of the promontories, look for the heron rookery made from two-by-fours.

At the clubhouse, cross over the trail that you started on and then continue straight ahead to the waterfall garden, featuring a maze of rocks and trees built up on a little hill. At the top of the hill, lake water is pumped out among the stands of Norway spruce, quaking aspen, and staghorn sumac before tumbling over four short waterfalls and through several shallow intermediate pools. From the base of the falls, the water runs along a brook back to the lake. On the backside of the waterfall, dozens of shrubs, trees, and ground-cover plants grow in the small conifer garden (look for the identification tags on individual plants). From the conifer garden, look for the paved road that runs next to the canal, and follow it away from the environmental learning center.

After you pass under Harlem Avenue Bridge, you'll see a series of waterfalls flowing over concrete embankments on the opposite side of the canal. This is one of five SEPA (sidestream elevated pool aeration) stations along the canal and the Little Calumet River. The SEPA stations clean the water by cooling it and increasing its oxygen content, while also providing a pleasant recreation area for local residents. Beyond the bridge, look for the small side trail leading to a bench overlooking the SEPA station.

After the SEPA station, you'll pass a mountain of wood chips and a couple of junctions on the right. Soon a clearing provides a nice view of the wooded banks across the channel. As the trail turns right, a small side trail leads to a bench with a view of the Ridgeland Avenue Bridge. Continuing to the right, follow the arrow pointing to the trail heading into the woods. Although this less-used trail may be slightly overgrown in spots with shrubs, it's still easy to follow. The trail occasionally becomes rugged and steep as it follows the rise and fall of a ridge running parallel to the canal on the right and IL 83 on the left.

Nearly halfway through the ridge hike, you'll encounter an overlook with a pavilion and benches. Among the trunks of cottonwood, elm, and hickory, you'll notice half-buried chunks of limestone. In 1955, when the Army Corp of Engineers widened the Cal–Sag Channel, they formed this ridge with the excavated earth and stone. At one point, the trail drops down sharply before it crosses an intermittent stream on a line of boulders. Continuing on, the trail grows wider and the surface becomes fuzzy with moss. Once you reach the open gravelly area, head back down to the trail on the side of the canal.

Just after passing under the bridge on the way back to the parking lot, take a left on the wide wood-chip trail. This trail leads to a boardwalk and a set of stairs and benches that winds through a wooded gully containing an intermittent stream. Following the stairs up the side of the gully brings you to the vegetable garden, complete with scarecrows and a variety of flowers and common vegetables. At the edge of the garden, a half-dozen pieces of old farm equipment are on display. From the vegetable garden, continue to the left through the small prairie and back to the parking lot.

■ TO THE TRAILHEAD

From Chicago, take I-55 southwest to Exit 283. Follow IL 43 (South Harlem Avenue) 8.4 miles to the left (south) to IL 83 (West College Drive). Turn right on IL 83 and proceed to the entrance of Lake Katherine Preserve, 0.3 miles ahead on the right.

Alternate directions from the northwest: Heading southeast on I-294, take the US 12/US 20 exit, heading east. Immediately turn right on IL 43, heading south for 3 miles to IL 83 (West College Drive). After turning right on IL 83, the entrance to the preserve is just ahead on the right.

Public transportation: Take the Orange CTA line to Midway Airport. At the Midway CTA station, take Pace Bus 386 to the corner of South Harlem Avenue and IL 83 (West College Drive). The entrance to Lake Katherine is a quarter mile west on West College Drive.

■ OVERVIEW

LENGTH: 2.5 miles

CONFIGURATION: 2 loops

SCENERY: Lake, oak woods, rolling terrain

EXPOSURE: Mostly shaded

SURFACE: Dirt with some gravel

HIKING TIME: 1.5–2 hours

ACCESS: March–October, 8 a.m.–5 p.m., weekends, 8 a.m.–5:30 p.m.; November–February, 8 a.m.– 4:30 p.m. Schoolhouse exhibit building opens at 9 a.m., closes a half hour earlier than the grounds and is closed Fridays. Also closed for major holidays.

FACILITIES: Water, restrooms

MAPS: Available in exhibit building; USGS topo Sag Bridge, IL

SPECIAL COMMENTS: No pets allowed on trails. The nature center offers educational programs year-round for kids and adults. This hike includes Farm Pond Trail, Black Oak Trail, and White Oak Trail. While the park map indicates that these trails measure 3 miles in all, my GPS device measured a total distance of 2.5 miles.

■ SNAPSHOT

With 2.5 miles of laid-back hiking and plenty of engaging exhibits, Little Red Schoolhouse Nature Center is particularly appealing for kids and beginning hikers. The trails run next to Long John Slough and through oak forests and savannas, as well as the occasional prairie.

■ UP CLOSE

When the first incarnation of the Little Red Schoolhouse opened its doors more than a century ago, it was a place where children from local farms learned the three R's. Over time, as the Palos Forest Preserve expanded, the school building was moved and eventually shut down. The schoolhouse and the grounds now serve as a place where adults and a new generation of kids can delve into the natural world—and receive a quick lesson on the history of rural education.

Inside the former one-room schoolhouse are taxidermy specimens of a coyote, a loon, an opossum, an assortment of birds, and a

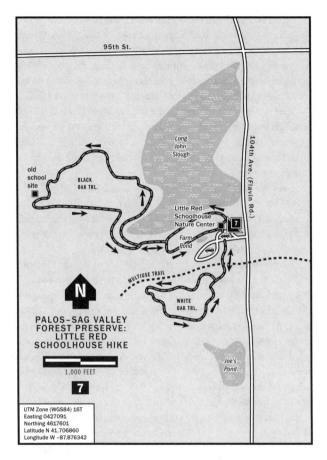

five-legged bullfrog named Mr. Lucky. More plentiful are the live animals, such as an American kestrel (a small falcon), a boisterous crow, and a variety of local frogs and snakes. A beehive covered in Plexiglas allows visitors a close view of bees in action. Mixed in with the nature exhibits are details about the old school. On display are photos and a diorama depicting life at the school when it was just to the west along what is now the Black Oak Trail.

Start on the Farm Pond Trail behind the nature center. From the nature center, the trail hugs the shore of Long John Slough, a 35-acre shallow lake fringed by cattails and oaks. During autumn and spring, the slough is a popular stop for migrating waterbirds. Between June and September, considerable sections of the slough are blanketed with lily pads and thousands of white water lilies.

At 0.2 miles, turn right at the fork to begin Black Oak Trail as it runs through a small restored prairie with grasses, sedges, and flowers. Passing beyond a gated fence, turn right again at a second fork. If hiking during summer, l listen for bullfrogs along the marshy edge of the slough.

As the trail turns away from the slough at a half mile, the woods become dense and quiet. The terrain flattens. Appearing regularly are trailside benches and folksy signs showing the animals and plants found in the preserve. Watch for black oaks, the trail's namesake, which possess jagged lobes on their leaves.

At 0.9 miles is a sign for the former site of the schoolhouse. First built here in 1870, the school burned to the ground in the mid-1880s and was quickly rebuilt. Life in the area began to change in 1915, when the forest preserve started acquiring many of the local farms. As families moved, the location of the schoolhouse was no longer convenient for many students. Shifting populations, combined with flooding problems on the site, prompted school officials to move the building in 1932. The forest preserve continued to expand, and the school was closed in 1948. In 1955, the school was moved to its present location and reopened as a nature center.

After passing the former school site, the trail follows the route of Old 99th Street. Beyond a marsh on the right at 1.2 miles is a short trail leading into a prairie. Nearby is an enclosure that park staff use to monitor the feeding habits of deer in the area. Finish the loop at 1.4 miles, and then head back through the gate, turning right to regain the Farm Pond Trail. At 1.6 miles, the trail ends at a display of old farm equipment. Be sure to check out the small, enclosed garden on the left, with a nice variety of native plants. Beyond the garden are three enormous cages containing a great horned owl, a barred owl, and a red-tailed hawk. Before moving on, swing toward the rear of the schoolhouse, where young hikers will enjoy watching the turtles in the small pool.

Even on busy weekends, when the Black Oak Trail and the nature center host a steady stream of visitors, you're still likely to find a quiet atmosphere on the White Oak Trail. Start the hike directly across the parking lot from the Little Red Schoolhouse. Just beyond a bench on the left overlooking a small pond, the trail crosses a multiuse path that runs through many sections of the 14,000-acre Palos–Sag Valley Forest Preserve. When you reach a fork at 0.2 miles, stay to the right as the path leads through lightly rolling terrain. Watch for woodpeckers, flickers, and Eastern bluebirds overhead. Joe's Pond, one of the many small bodies of water in the area left behind by glaciers, is visible through the trees on the right at 0.6 miles. As the trail turns back toward the schoolhouse, there's a small ravine to the right. Lush with plants, it's a favorite spot for deer during the summer. Complete the loop at 0.8 miles and head back to the parking lot.

■ TO THE TRAILHEAD

Heading south from Chicago, take I-55 to Exit 279A. Follow La Grange Road (US 12, US 20) south for 3.5 miles. Turn right (west) on 95th Street. Follow 95th Street for 1.25 miles, turning left (south) on 104th Avenue (Flavin Road). Little Red Schoolhouse Nature Center is on the right, a half mile south of 95th Street.

■ MORE FUN

Outdoor explorers in the Chicago area are lucky to have the massive Palos–Sag Valley Forest Preserve in their midst. Within thousands of acres of hilly woodland, rolling prairie, and scenic wetlands are some 35 miles of multiuse trails and many more miles of narrow unmarked side trails. In the past several years, the Cook County Forest Preserve District has made exploring at Palos and Sag Valley easier by color-coding the major trails, marking major intersections, and installing confidence markers on the trails. Find out about all the hiking and biking options at the forest preserves by visiting **www.fpdcc.com.**

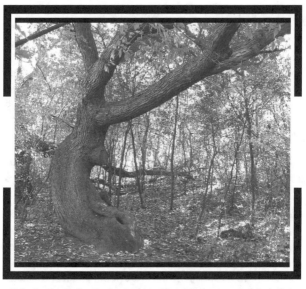

Native American trail-marker trees—such as this one that appears along the trail at
Bristol Woods—usually pointed to an important local destination.

North Chicagoland
and Wisconsin

OVERVIEW

LENGTH: 2.6 miles	**ACCESS:** 7 a.m.–10 p.m.
CONFIGURATION: Combo	**FACILITIES:** Picnic tables, shelter, toilets, playground
SCENERY: Oak and bottomland woods, marshes, pond, nature center, old town hall	**MAPS:** Available in the nature center; USGS topo Paddock Lake, WI
EXPOSURE: Shaded	**SPECIAL COMMENTS:** The nature center is open Tuesday–Sunday, 9 a.m.–4 p.m. Contact the nature center at (262) 857-8008 or visit www.pringlenc.org for more information.
SURFACE: Dirt, grass	
HIKING TIME: 1 hour	

SNAPSHOT

At Bristol Woods, hikers will enjoy the pleasantly rolling terrain covered in bottomland forest and oak woodland. Tree connoisseurs will enjoy the many oak specimens of considerable size, as well as a rare Native American trail-marker tree.

UP CLOSE

Once owned by a local parks commissioner, Bristol Woods offers visitors a pleasant stroll through nearly 200 acres of upland and lowland woods sprinkled with small marshes. The park came into existence in the 1970s when the county bought most of the property at a bargain price from Bob Pringle Sr., a one-time farmer who then served on the Kenosha County Parks Commission. Around the same time, the Pringle family also donated money toward the construction of a nature center. Now operated by volunteers from the Hoy chapter of the Audubon Society in Racine, the Pringle Nature Center has a nice collection of mounted birds and animals as well as habitat exhibits.

Starting the hike behind the nature center, you'll immediately come upon a tree with a strange crescent-shaped trunk. This

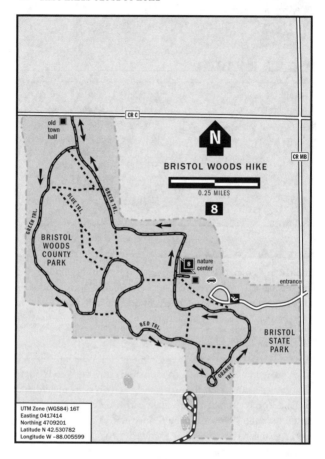

BRISTOL WOODS HIKE

0.25 MILES

8

old town hall

GREEN TRL.

BLUE TRL.

GREEN TRL.

BRISTOL WOODS COUNTY PARK

8 nature center

entrance

RED TRL.

ORANGE TRL.

BRISTOL STATE PARK

CR C

CR MB

UTM Zone (WGS84) 16T
Easting 0417414
Northing 4709201
Latitude N 42.530782
Longitude W −88.005599

200-year-old oak is one of the last Native American trail-marker trees in Kenosha County. While this tree is slightly different, most trail-marker trees were created by stripping a sapling of its branches and then bending it to the ground in the direction of any number of important locations, such as camping or trading areas, sacred spots, or natural springs. Once a branch appeared on the top side in the middle of the bent trunk, this branch was allowed to grow skyward. The weight of the branch ensured that the trunk stayed bent. Later, the trunk beyond the lone vertical branch was removed. While this trail-marker tree lines up nicely with the existing trail, no one is certain what it originally pointed toward.

Just ahead, at the T-junction on the edge of a small marsh, turn right. Turn right again on the Red Trail (trails are marked with colored posts at nearly all junctions). Heading down a gradual incline, you'll pass by the little cattail pond in the open space in front of the nature center. Stay to the left as a grassy trail runs to the right toward the open area. The trail crosses an intermittent stream before it rises and runs through a small ravine filled with hickory, oak, and walnut trees. The terrain becomes more rolling as the trail swings left and then zigzags alongside the agricultural field on the right (keep an eye out for deer in the field). The trail eventually drops down a steep slope and heads through a small ravine strewn with deadfall.

After turning right at the Green Trail, the path guides you along a raised bed with a crushed gravel surface. An attractive bottomland forest appears on the right, and a steep hill rises up on the left. Stay to the right and switch to the Blue Trail as it rises gradually toward the old town hall located on County Road C. A sign in front of the white wood-frame building explains that it was built in 1870 and actively used for the next 100 years. As you backtrack along the blue trail, skip the first trail that heads toward the back of the town hall. Instead, take the second right, the Green Trail, which leads through a small clearing with a picnic table and then climbs before taking a couple of banked turns.

Passing the White Trail on the left, you'll see more agricultural land through the trees on the right. From here, the trail makes a long and gradual descent under a canopy of large, eye-catching oaks. Watch for downy woodpeckers gliding between the specimens of bur, red, white, and black oak. Heading away from the agricultural field, the trail starts to drop. You may notice that the sides of this trail, as well as other trails at Bristol Woods, contain a good number of rocks and modest-sized boulders. Dropped off by the last glacier, these rocks were usually removed by farmers so they wouldn't damage their plows. The abundance of rocks at Bristol Woods reveals that this area was never farmed; it was one of the few natural areas in the Chicago region to escape the plow. Just after the trail takes a sharp left turn at a large white oak, keep straight ahead on the Green Trail as you pass an unmarked trail on the right that connects with the Red Trail.

Arriving at a cluster of cottonwood and elm trees, turn right on the Red Trail as it leads past a bench. After a few turns and a series of intermittent streams, you'll see a marker at a grouping of cedars, followed by another intermittent stream that runs through a small gully. After the junction with the Yellow Trail, you'll pass a couple of huge white oaks and then climb a bit before arriving at a bench situated under another cluster of cedars on a little hilltop. From the hill, walk down into a shallow ravine and then cross an intermittent stream that has carved out a rocky trough. A short climb brings you to a junction with the unmarked connector trail on the right; nearby you'll see a wall from a foundation of a former barn.

After a stretch of bottomland forest thick with bushes, you'll encounter another junction with a connector trail, as well as a marsh behind the trees on the left. Following a dense section of trail that is almost tunnel-like, turn right on the Orange Trail. Stay to the right and you'll see more marshland through the trees on the right. Complete the loop and then head back to the Red Trail.

Back on the Red Trail, look for a grove of apple trees that were once part of a nearby farm. After passing a trail on the right that goes toward the park road, the trail leads you into a little ravine containing a grove of quaking aspen. This final section of the trail brings you beside several monster-sized oaks, some with knotty, arthritic-looking limbs. Turn right on the Yellow Trail and then bear left back to the nature center.

■ TO THE TRAILHEAD

Follow I-90/I-94 northwest from Chicago. Stay on I-94 as it breaks off and follow it 45 miles north. Two miles into Wisconsin, take

Exit 347, County Road Q. Turn left (west) and proceed for 2.5 miles until you reach County Road MB. Turn right (north) on CR MB and proceed 0.4 miles. The entrance to the park is on the left.

■ MORE FUN

West of Bristol Woods is Silver Lake County Park, which offers several miles of hilly trails running above the lake through groves of oak and sumac and pine plantations. Catch the beginning of the loop from the small parking area just inside the park entrance. Turning left on the park road at the entrance brings you to a lake-side picnic area. Taking the road to the right brings you through a number of picnic areas sprinkled throughout the pleasantly hilly park. The park is open from 7 a.m. to 10 p.m. From Bristol Woods, take County Road MB left (north) to IL 50. Follow IL 50 left (west) for 6 miles to County Road F. Turn left (south) on CR F, and the park entrance is nearly 2 miles ahead on the right.

9   Glacial Park Loop

■ OVERVIEW

LENGTH: 5 miles

CONFIGURATION: 2 connected loops with 1 brief out-and-back segment

SCENERY: Savannas, prairies, a marsh, a bog, a creek, and expansive views from high spots

EXPOSURE: Mostly open

SURFACE: Hard-packed dirt, mowed grass, and wood chips

HIKING TIME: 2.5–3 hours

ACCESS: Sunrise–sunset

FACILITIES: Picnic areas, restrooms, water, sledding hill, and canoe launch

MAPS: Available at trail boards at the parking areas; USGS topo Richmond, IL

SPECIAL COMMENTS: For information on activities at the park such as the Trail of History event and cross-country skiing, call the McHenry County Conservation District at (815) 338-6223.

■ SNAPSHOT

While hiking the trails of Glacial Park Conservation Area, you'll glide through open prairies, meander beside a lovely creek, and bound over hills that undulate like ocean waves. The star attraction, though, is a collection of curious mounds left by a receding glacier.

■ UP CLOSE

For those with an interest in learning the ways in which glaciers sculpted the landscape in northeastern Illinois, Glacial Park is a geologic jewel. The most eye-catching landforms in the park are mounds—called kames—that are formed when glacial meltwater deposits heaps of sand and gravel in depressions in the ice or at the edge of the glacier. The 100-foot-high Camelback Kame, which this hike passes over, is said to have formed at the edge of a glacier as it receded 15,500 years ago. The park's bog and marshes also offer a visual link to the area's geologic past. These wetlands began to take shape when large chunks of ice detached from a receding glacier. As ice melted, a pond formed in the depression, and eventually vegetation overtook the pond.

But it's not just the geologic heritage that lends appeal to this 2,800-acre park: its variety—as well as its beauty and tranquility—make it a splendid place to stretch your legs and get a concentrated dose of the natural world. Start the hike from the west side of the Wiedrich Education Center parking lot. Taking the trail on the right, marked by the sign for the Deerpath, Coyote, and Nippersink trails, you'll enter a rolling prairie fringed by oaks. After passing a small amphitheatre built into the hillside with large stone blocks, turn right at the first intersection. At a quarter mile into the hike, the trail leaves the prairie and enters an oak savanna where the landscape begins to rise and fall in various directions. At 0.4 miles, take in a great view of the prairie, marshland, and creek to the west.

After the overlook, the path runs beneath a canopy of gnarled oak limbs as it descends from the hilltop. Following a hairpin turn to the right, the path rises toward the Camelback

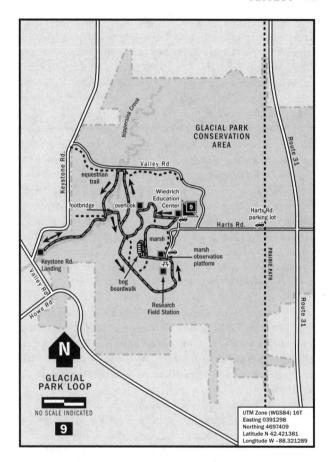

Kame. Stay to the right at the next two trail junctions, and then head down the hill, saving the hike up the kame for the return trip. Turn right again at 0.8 miles into the hike after passing through the metal gate. From here, it's a straight walk to a small glacial kame alongside Valley Road.

While hiking along this trail, keep an eye out over the prairie for the northern harrier, a medium-sized hawk that is fun to watch as it hunts for its prey by cruising close to the ground above grasslands and marshes (another way to identify this frequent visitor to the park is by a clearly visible white spot on its rump). Once you reach the small kame, you'll have a better view of two more kames on the other side of the road. Follow Valley Road left as it crosses Nippersink Creek, and then turn left again on the horse-and-snowmobile trail that heads back on the other side of the creek.

At the junction near the footbridge, keep straight ahead as the path comes alongside this twisting section of the creek. Continue ahead on this pleasant streamside path until you reach the Keystone Road Landing, where you'll find an observation platform at the edge of the creek, as well as a picnic area, a canoe launch, and restrooms. The wetlands on the other side of the creek contain one of the Nippersink's many local feeder streams. The presence of these feeder streams account for the Nippersink's name, which means "place of small waters" in the Algonquin language. From the landing, retrace your steps back to the footbridge. After crossing the bridge, you'll enter a large mowed area at the base of Camelback Kame.

Each year in mid-October, the park hosts a large event in this spot called the Trail of History. Through exhibits, demonstrations, and people dressed in traditional costumes, visitors get a glimpse of life for early European settlers in the area. The wigwam frames on the eastern shore of the creek and a nearby cabin serve as exhibits for this event.

At 3.3 miles, pass through the gate again, head up the hill, and turn right to ascend the spine of the Camelback Kame, named for its gentle double hump. Kames can be cone-shaped, like the ones by Valley Road, or they can be ridgelike, such as the Camelback. These glacial deposits are somewhat rare in the region, largely because many of them have been carted away for their sand and gravel.

As you descend the kame, continue straight ahead at the next two trail junctions. Soon the trail leaves the prairie and enters a savanna. On the left you'll see the park's research field station. At 4.3 miles into the hike, just before reaching the main parking lot, follow the trail left as it runs through a picnic area. After crossing the park road, proceed straight ahead alongside a large marsh. First, however, you may want to take a short detour to an observation deck on the right.

When you cross the Deerpath Trail at 4.6 miles into the hike, continue ahead, following the sign for a bog boardwalk. The bog is dominated by leatherleaf, a shrub that keeps its leaves all year round. Finishing the short boardwalk, follow the loop that brings you back up to the Deerpath Trail, where you'll turn left. After the trail takes a steep drop, keep straight ahead at the next junction, and then turn left at another junction, heading up the hill and back to the Wiedrich Education Center parking lot.

■ TO THE TRAILHEAD

From Chicago, head north on I-90/I-94. Follow I-94 as it separates from I-90. Continue on I-94 until you reach West Belvidere Road (IL 120). Turn left (west) on Belvidere Road and follow it for 18 miles until you reach IL 31 (North Richmond Road). Turn right (north) on IL 31 and travel 6 miles. Turn left (west) on Harts Road and follow the signs for 1 mile until you reach the Wiedrich Education Center.

■ MORE FUN

After entering the park on Harts Road, look for a parking lot for the Prairie Trail, a 25.9-mile multiuse path that stretches from the Wisconsin border south to Kane County. Once in Kane County, the Prairie Trail connects with a couple of other long trails: the Fox River Trail and the Illinois Prairie Path.

■ OVERVIEW

LENGTH: 2.1 miles

CONFIGURATION: Loop, with a spur leading to the beach

SCENERY: River, marshes, savanna, beach, dunes, Lake Michigan

EXPOSURE: Mostly exposed

SURFACE: Dirt, sand

HIKING TIME: 1 hour

ACCESS: Sunrise–8 p.m.

FACILITIES: Restrooms, water

MAPS: Available at the nature center; USGS topo Zion, IL

SPECIAL COMMENTS: In recent years, asbestos has washed up on the beach at this park. After rounds of testing, the state of Illinois and the U.S. Environmental Protection Agency maintain that the beach is not a health hazard.

Pets must be leashed. Large crowds descend upon the park for events on various spring and summer weekends. Call the park at (847) 662-4811 for exact dates. The park office is open Tuesday–Saturday, 8 a.m.–4 p.m. The park's Web site is accessible from www.dnr.state.il.us.

■ SNAPSHOT

After a ramble along the shore of the Dead River, this trail brings you through some of the only sand dunes left in the state of Illinois. Halfway through the hike, take a break on a surprisingly quiet stretch of Lake Michigan beach.

■ UP CLOSE

While it's true that Illinois Beach State Park is one of the most popular beaches in the region, it's also true that visitors rarely seem to step away from the main beach and picnic area, leaving the trails and the out-of-the-way beach on this hike surprisingly quiet. The park consists of two separate areas, referred to as the northern unit and southern unit. The southern unit, where this hike takes place, is the larger section, with more amenities, such as a campground, a store, and even a resort and conference center.

Catch the beginning of Dead River Trail near the far end of the parking lot. After you hike 0.2 miles through oak savanna, the

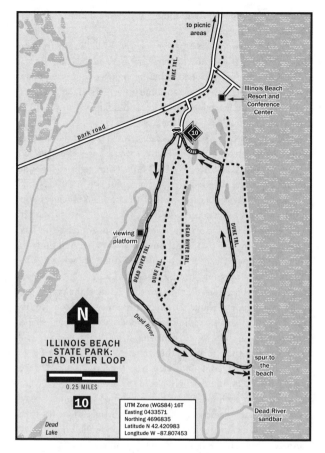

to picnic
areas

BIKE TRL.

park road

Illinois Beach
Resort and
Conference
Center

10

viewing
platform

DEAD RIVER TRL.

DUNE TRL.

DEAD RIVER TRL.

DUNE TRL.

Dead River

N

**ILLINOIS BEACH
STATE PARK:
DEAD RIVER LOOP**

0.25 MILES

10

spur to
the
beach

Dead River
sandbar

Dead
Lake

UTM Zone (WGS84) 16T
Easting 0433571
Northing 4696835
Latitude N 42.420983
Longitude W −87.807453

trail meets up with the marshy waterway known as the Dead
River. If you have the impression that this looks more like a long
pond than a river, you're right; this river only flows during certain
times of the year when the water levels rise. Most of the year
a sandbar blocks the mouth at Lake Michigan, thus keeping the
water contained. Another 0.2 miles ahead is a platform overlooking
the river and the expansive wetland. Some geologists have said the

once-sluggish Chicago River looked much like the Dead River in pre-settlement times.

While the water here may be at a standstill, the environment certainly is not. During the spring, summer, and into fall, the trail hosts a variety of wildflowers, including milkweeds, shooting stars, and gentians. You're likely to see some waterbirds in the river, and, if visiting during the winter after snow has fallen, you might see a network of animal tracks on the ice.

Shortly after passing a kitchen stove–sized boulder in the middle of the stream, the trail turns toward Lake Michigan and the scenery starts to change. At 0.7 miles, turn right at the junction. Leaving the wooded stream bank and oak savanna, you'll enter a washboard landscape made of sand. Because the prevailing winds blow the sand out to the lake, these are low dunes with gentle slopes. Each line of dunes was a previous shoreline for Lake Michigan during the past few thousand years. Here and there the dunes are topped with scrawny oak trees that struggle to gather nutrients from the sandy ground. In all, an impressive 650 species of plants have been identified in the south unit of the park. Some of the low creeping plants to look for among the dunes are the bearberry, with small paddle-shaped leaves and little egg-shaped white flowers, and the Waukegan juniper, an evergreen with whitish berries that turn purple in the winter.

The lake will come into view near the junction at 1.2 miles into the hike. Continue straight ahead to a stretch of beach where you're likely to encounter few people, even on hot summer days. For a short beach stroll, walk 0.2 miles to the right to see the sandbar at the mouth of the Dead River. One-and-a-half miles to the south you'll see the Commonwealth Edison coal-fired generating plant, and 2.5 miles to the north is the Zion nuclear power plant, which provides electricity for much of the Chicago area. Dedicated beach ramblers can follow the beach north for 0.7 miles to catch the trail back to the parking lot.

To continue on the hiking route, head back up to the main trail and take a right. While walking parallel to the lake, one will see water between the swells of sand. At the base of the mounds, look for miniature blowouts where the wind has scoured away the plants and created hollow spots. As the trail bends inland, the oak trees grow larger and the landscape becomes blanketed in grasses typical of savannas and prairies. At 1.9 miles into the hike, turn left at the junction, and then pass a large marsh on the right before following a boardwalk for 30 yards over a shallow dune pond. From the boardwalk, the parking lot is a short distance straight ahead.

■ TO THE TRAILHEAD

Follow I-90/I-94 northwest from Chicago. Stay on I-94 as it breaks off, and follow it north for 35 miles. Exit at Grand Avenue (IL 132) and go east for 3.5 miles. Then turn left (north) on Green Bay Road (IL 131). Proceed north 4 miles before turning right (east) on Wadsworth Road. Follow Wadsworth Road for 3 miles into the park. Stay to the right and park in the second parking area on the right.

Public transportation: Take the Union Pacific–North Metra Line to Zion. From the Zion station, the trailhead is a 3-mile walk or bike ride, primarily along pathways. Head south on the path that runs on the west side of the train tracks. Turn left (east) on 29th Street and then continue straight on the paved path as the road turns left. Follow the path as it snakes along the beach, heads inland, and arrives at the parking area.

■ MORE FUN

If you're looking for a picnic area and a lively—sometimes crowded—stretch of beach, you're in luck. Just continue ahead on the park road, past the hotel on the right. Illinois Beach State Park also offers a campground containing 244 sites, many of which are fairly close to the beach.

Several more miles of hiking trails can be found in the northern unit of the park. To reach the northern unit, leave the park the way you entered via Wadsworth Road. After the train tracks, turn right (north) on Sheridan Road. Turn right (east) on 17th Street and stay to the left. Pick up the trail near the circle turnaround at the end of the road.

OVERVIEW

LENGTH: 4.5 miles	**FACILITIES:** Water, restrooms, visitor center
CONFIGURATION: Loop within a loop	**MAPS:** Trail maps available at the visitor center; USGS topo Wheeling, IL
SCENERY: Lush forest along Des Plaines River	
EXPOSURE: Shady, with brief exposed stretches	**SPECIAL COMMENTS:** The visitor center is open 9 a.m.–5 p.m. daily, except major holidays. Ryerson Woods is open 6:30 a.m.–sunset. No pets or picnicking allowed. Visit www.ryersonwoods.org to learn about Ryerson's plants and animals and programs offered throughout the year.
SURFACE: Dirt with numerous boardwalks and bridges	
HIKING TIME: 3–4 hours for both loops	
ACCESS: 6:30 a.m.–sunset	

SNAPSHOT

The trails in Ryerson Woods wind through some of the most stunning forestland in the Chicago region. Along the shore of the Des Plaines River and its backwater, expect to see waterfowl, wildflowers, and old rustic cabins left behind by the families that once owned the property.

UP CLOSE

What was a once a weekend getaway for a local industrialist and his friends is now a hikers' heaven, with trails leading through one of the finest woodlands in Northern Illinois. Much of what is now the south section of Ryerson Woods was purchased in the 1920s by Edward L. Ryerson and his friends. Ryerson, who became president of Ryerson Steel Company upon the death of his father in 1928, built a rustic cabin on his riverside plot. In years to come, his friends also built cabins on the land. In 1938, Ryerson bought 250 acres of farmland in what is now the northern section of the conservation area, and then a few years later he built a summer home that now serves as park offices. Motivated by a desire to maintain this forest

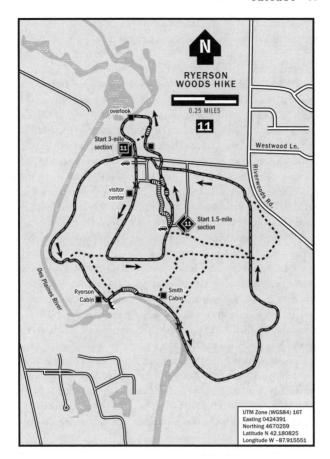

RYERSON
WOODS HIKE

0.25 MILES

11

overlook

Start 3-mile
section

11

Westwood Ln.

visitor
center

Riverwoods Rd.

Start 1.5-mile
section

11

Des Plaines River

Ryerson
Cabin

Smith
Cabin

UTM Zone (WGS84) 16T
Easting 0424391
Northing 4670259
Latitude N 42.180825
Longitude W –87.915551

sanctuary, in the 1960s Ryerson and his friends decided to donate
and sell their land to the Lake County Forest Preserve District.

Given Ryerson Woods' startling beauty and its proximity
to Chicago, one would expect it to be swarming with hikers and
nature watchers. Fortunately, this is not the case. Perhaps it's the
restrictions on pets, bicycles, and picnicking that keep the crowds
away. Despite the lack of traditional park amenities, Ryerson is still

a great place to bring the family. At the farm exhibit in the north section of the preserve, kids will enjoy the pigs, goats, chickens, cows, beehives, and turkeys. Also, the layout of trails allows for easy shortening or lengthening of a hike.

Map boards are posted at trailheads and at a handful of trail intersections. Picking up a map from the visitor center will ensure that you always know where you are. The first part of this hike, which starts at the parking area near the Brushwood House, takes you on a 1.5-mile loop through the northern section of the preserve. The second part of the hike, which starts near the farm and visitor center, takes you on a 3-mile loop more or less along the perimeter of the preserve. Catch the beginning of the hike's first part just left of the driveway that leads into the parking lot near the Brushwood House. Right away on the trail, on the right, you'll notice a high fence, which allows Ryerson Woods staff to monitor the amount of browsing done by deer.

At about 0.2 miles, near a couple of boardwalks spanning intermittent streams, you'll get a taste of what makes the Ryerson Woods landscape so beautiful: tall oaks, hickories, elms, dense canopies, minimal understory, and a lush, leafy ground cover. Coming out of the woods, the trail takes a sharp right turn as it begins to run alongside a park road that borders the farm property. Keep going on this mowed path, passing the intersection with the perimeter loop trail and then crossing the park entrance road. In the clearing across the road, keep an eye out for bluebirds and indigo buntings, and—if it's dusk—for the bats leaving the bat house. The trail continues to the left, running between the two cabins, which are used for programs and exhibits when school groups visit.

At the next junction, turn right and cross a boardwalk. After you walk through a grove of large shagbark hickories and cross a bridge next to a couple of sizable oaks, the Des Plaines River will appear on the right. In a short distance, you'll find a bench at a modest overlook of the river. After the overlook, take the next trail to the right, which takes you back to the park entrance road. The hike continues on the other side of a parking lot and the farm building in front of you. Before getting back to the trail, you may want to stroll around the farm to see the livestock. Although Edward Ryerson kept dairy cattle and Yorkshire pigs, his main interest was Arabian horses, which were kept in these structures designed by Edwin Hill Clark, the architect who designed the famous Brookfield Zoo in Brookfield, Illinois.

Back on the trail, you'll cross a bridge and enter the forest. In this area and in others, don't be alarmed at seeing garbage bags on the trail waiting to be picked up. Most likely the bags contain an invasive, quickly spreading plant called mustard garlic, which has been pulled up by volunteers. Turn left at the T-intersection and continue along this wide, gravelly path until you come to a trail that branches left. Follow this short trail through an open area and back to the parking lot.

Pick up the 3-mile perimeter hike at the parking lot by the farm and the visitor center. Starting in the corner of the parking lot closest to the woods, this trail traverses the edges of the open space for a quarter mile, and then rambles alongside the backwater of the Des Plaines River. During spring and summer, watch for trilliums as well as irises, which are called blue flags and yellow flags. At about 0.4 miles into the hike, as the trail approaches the main thread of the river, consider slowing your pace: it's a favorite place for great blue herons. In the low spots, receding water has left logs strewn about.

Stay to the right at the intersection, and at 0.9 miles you'll reach Ryerson Cabin and a small dam in the river. From the back-right corner of the cabin, continue with the trail as it runs along the bank of the river and over a boardwalk that protects the softer, erosion-prone areas of the riverbank. Ahead is the intersection with another trail and the Smith Cabin, as well as a bench and a map board. Beyond the Smith Cabin, cross a bridge over a twisting stream, and head back into the forest. If rain has recently fallen, hikers in Ryerson Woods should expect to get mud on their shoes, particularly on this section of the trail, as it weaves among small marshes and intermittent ponds. After crossing the stream again, you'll pass through groves of elms, patches of mayapples, and towering oaks.

At 2.3 miles you'll see a map board and a bench at a trail intersection. Continue straight through more-dense woodland and marshy areas with boardwalks. The path turns left just before reaching a metal gate and soon runs alongside the park entrance road. A short way up, pass a trail intersection on the left and come out on the road that borders the farm area. Return to the parking lot by following the road on the right to the other side of the farm.

■ TO THE TRAILHEAD

From Chicago, head north on I-90/I-94. Follow I-94 as it separates from I-90. Continue on I-94 to Deerfield Road. Turn left (west) on Deerfield Road and proceed a half mile. At Riverwoods Road, turn right (north). Two miles ahead, turn left at the sign for the Edward L. Ryerson Conservation Area.

Public transportation: Ryerson is a 3.5-mile bike ride from both the Deerfield station on the Milwaukee District–North Metra Line and the Buffalo Grove station on the North Central Service Metra Line. See the Active Transportation Alliance's "Chicagoland Bicycle Map" for good routes between Ryerson and these stations.

12 Chicago Botanic Garden Hike

■ OVERVIEW

LENGTH: 2.7 miles	**FACILITIES:** Visitor center, cafe, restrooms, gift shop, library, ATM, wheelchairs, and telephones
CONFIGURATION: Large loop with a few short loops attached	
	MAPS: Pick up a map at the visitor center; USGS topo Highland Park, IL
SCENERY: Islands, prairie, oak woodland, marsh, and acres of pristine gardens	**SPECIAL COMMENTS:** No pets allowed. Two different tram tours run seasonally. Tickets and information are available at the booth outside of the visitor center. Check out www.chicagobotanic.org for more information.
EXPOSURE: Mostly exposed	
SURFACE: Paved, gravel, wood chips	
HIKING TIME: 1 hour	
ACCESS: 8 a.m.–sunset, except Christmas Day. Garden is free; parking is $15/car.	

■ S N A P S H O T

If you love to see carefully selected flowers, trees, and bushes grow-ing in perfectly landscaped environments, the Chicago Botanic Garden is a slice of heaven. While the interior gardens are justifi-ably the main attraction here, many visitors miss the additional gardens, the prairie and woodland, and the striking views that accompany a walk through the outer perimeter of the garden, high-lighted in this hike.

■ U P   C L O S E

Among the Botanic Garden's 305 acres of artfully landscaped grounds, there are 23 distinct gardens, including Japanese- and English-style gardens, rose and bulb gardens, fruit and vegetable gardens, and gardens specially designed for children and for wheel-chair access. Along with this excess of gardens, there are attractive bridges, statues, fountains, and plenty of scenic spots situated among the nine islands and the surrounding shoreline. Owned by the Cook County Forest Preserve District and managed by the Chicago Horticultural Society, the gardens are just part of what goes on here. The Botanic Garden has programs in education and research and offers a number of special events and services, such as classes, plant sales, opportunities to consult master gardeners, con-certs, and speakers.

From the visitor center, start the hike by heading straight across the North Lawn to the service road leading over the lake at the far end of the garden. On the other side of the bridge, pine trees grow on the left and buckeye trees on the right. Take either the ser-vice road or the narrow, paved path to the left. In the lake is Spider Island, thick with alders, birch, and serviceberry trees. On the right, the Skokie River runs along the bottom of a shallow ravine. Also on the right are a newly added brick wall and 1,600 new tree plantings intended to block noise and pollution from I-94. Extending from Spider Island to the serpentine-shaped bridge that leads to Evening Island is the Sensory Garden, which hosts plants and trees that pro-duce an array of colors, sounds, fragrances, and textures.

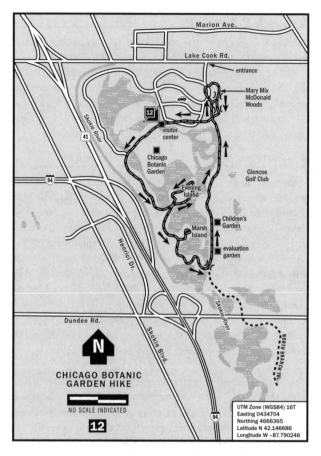

Marion Ave.

Lake Cook Rd.

entrance

Mary Mix
McDonald
Woods

12

visitor
center

Chicago
Botanic
Garden

Skokie River

41

94

Evening
Island

Glencoe
Golf Club

Marsh
Island

Children's
Garden

evaluation
garden

Skokie River

Henrici Dr.

Dundee Rd.

Skokie Blvd.

NORTH BRANCH TRL.

N

**CHICAGO BOTANIC
GARDEN HIKE**

NO SCALE INDICATED

12

94

UTM Zone (WGS84) 16T
Easting 0434704
Northing 4666365
Latitude N 42.146686
Longitude W –87.790246

Just ahead on the left, take the gravel trail to Evening Island,
added to the botanic garden in 2002 at a cost of $16 million. In
gardening circles, the design of this 5-acre island is called the "new
American" garden style and is inspired by landscapes such as the
meadow and the Midwestern prairie. As you climb the hill in the
center of the island, watch how the placement of trees nicely frames
the views of the nearby shoreline and prairie. Near the top of the

hill, a circle of large stones provides a great place to relax. The square metal tower, called a carillon, contains 48 bronze bells that weigh between 24 pounds and 2.5 tons (check in at the visitor center for information on regular carillon concerts). The bridges on the north side of the island provide a connection with the main gardens and complete the outline of a section of the lake called the Great Basin.

Back on the paved road, pass a few burr oak trees and several purple-martin houses attached to poles as you head into the 15-acre prairie. Entering the prairie, take the gravel trail left, and stay left at the next couple of junctions before crossing a bridge for a quick tour of Marsh Island. Botanic Garden staff maintains that Marsh Island (actually a wet prairie) is the best location on the grounds for spotting waterbirds and songbirds. Coming off Marsh Island, stay left as you pass a section of hilly prairie on the right—the dry, rocky soil is the reason that the grass is shorter at the top of the hill compared to the sides and bottom. After the small hills, take your pick of following the paved road, the dirt path, or the paved path, all of which lead to the bridge. On the way to the bridge, you'll pass compass plants (tall yellow flowers) and more burr oaks.

The bridge divides the Botanic Garden lake on the left and the Skokie River on the right. On the other side of the bridge, turn left on the paved road and pass the plant-production area, which grows 420,000 plants annually. Next on the right is the Children's Garden, where kids can get involved in activities such as watering plants, digging in soil, and climbing through a plant maze. The garden on the left contains roses that are evaluated for qualities such as color, fragrance, novelty, and vigor. The next garden, featuring a big sundial surrounded by 7,000 herbaceous plants, also serves as an evaluation garden. Both of these evaluation gardens keep out deer by using solar-powered electric fencing that is turned on after hours.

After you pass a stand of downy-hawthorn trees next to the road, three islands come into view, each carefully landscaped and pruned in traditional Japanese styles. A low zigzag bridge connects the first and second islands. Off in the distance, between the second and third islands, a waterfall tumbles some 45 feet over granite boulders. The inaccessible third island contains smaller trees that are intended to present the optical illusion that the island is far off in the distance.

Finish the hike with a brief stroll through the Mary Mix McDonald Woods, the only location at the Botanic Garden where the soil is undisturbed. Enter the oak woodland on the right before the road curves to the left. Stay to the left on the path as you pass over a series of footbridges spanning intermittent streams and several boardwalks. Along this path there's a steady progression of signs identifying plants and animals of the area and describing the basic concepts of woodland restoration in northeastern Illinois. Because this trail crosses the park road, watch for traffic, especially on the weekends. In a number of spots you'll see that the Botanic Garden is engaged in a serious fencing campaign to keep deer out of the area. When finished with the hike through the McDonald Woods, continue along the paved road to the parking lots just ahead. Or if you wish to return to the visitor center or explore more of the interior gardens, follow the wood-chip path that runs parallel to the lake and take the service road left to the visitor center.

■ TO THE TRAILHEAD

Follow I-90/I-94 northwest, continuing on I-94 for 13.5 miles after I-90 splits off. At Exit 29, remain on the Edens Expressway (US 41); then take the next exit for Lake Cook Road. Turn right (east) and travel for a half mile to the Botanic Garden. Follow signs to the parking areas.

Public transportation: Save yourself the $15 parking fee and take the Metra. The Union Pacific–North Metra Line stops within a mile of the Botanic Garden. On Sundays during the warmer months, take Metra to the Glencoe station, and then take the Garden Trolley to the Botanic Garden (for trains arriving/departing from 9:30 a.m. to 5 p.m. at the Glencoe station). You can also walk to the garden from the Braeside Metra station (head west for nearly 1 mile along Lake Cook Road to the garden entrance). From Davis Street, Glencoe, and Highland Park Metra stations, take bus 213 to the garden.

Bicycle: Three long bike trails run into or near the Botanic Garden. To the east is Green Bay Trail, to the west is the southern terminus of the Skokie Valley Bikeway, and coming from the south is the ever-popular North Branch Trail, which brings you right into the garden's grounds.

■ MORE FUN

At the southern edge of the Chicago Botanic Garden, visitors can connect with the 20.1-mile North Branch Trail. One of the great urban pathways of Chicagoland, the North Branch Trail runs through the Skokie Lagoons and along the North Branch of the Chicago River. To reach the trail from the botanic garden, head south on the service road on the east side of the lake. The path starts on the other side of Dundee Road.

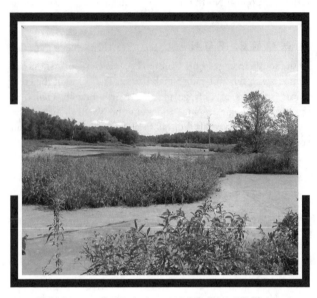

Wetlands cover much of the landscape at LaSalle Fish and Wildlife Area.

South Chicagoland and Indiana

■ OVERVIEW

LENGTH: 3.3 miles	**ACCESS:** 8 a.m.–sunset
CONFIGURATION: Combo	**FACILITIES:** Picnic tables and shelters, visitor center, restrooms
SCENERY: Bottomland forest, marshland, oak woodland, Little Calumet River, a 19th-century working farm, and an early trader's homestead	**MAPS:** Available at the map board and in the visitor center; USGS topo Chesterton, IN
EXPOSURE: All shaded, except through the prairie	**SPECIAL COMMENTS:** The Chellberg Farmhouse and the Bailly Homestead are open May–October on Sundays. Learn more by visiting www.nps.gov/indu.
SURFACE: Dirt, grass	
HIKING TIME: 2 hours	

■ SNAPSHOT

Get a glimpse of early settlement life in northwestern Indiana by touring the homesteads of two frontier families. You'll also see wooded ravines, rich bottomland forest that grows beside the Little Calumet River, and a curious old cemetery.

■ UP CLOSE

The Indiana Dunes are chock-full of scenic vistas and appealing places to explore. Throughout the area, more than a half-dozen trail systems offer hikes ranging in length from a half mile to 10 miles and up. Trails run through prairies and woods, they run along the beaches, and they ascend some of the highest dunes on the south shore of Lake Michigan. While you won't run into any monster-sized dunes on this hike, you will find woods, prairie, and creeks nestled within an alluring landscape. You'll also come across an assortment of historic attractions that help us imagine what the surrounding area was like before it became the hub of heavy industry that it is today.

In 1874, ten years after emigrating from Sweden, Anders and Johanna Chellberg were farming 80 acres within a growing Swedish

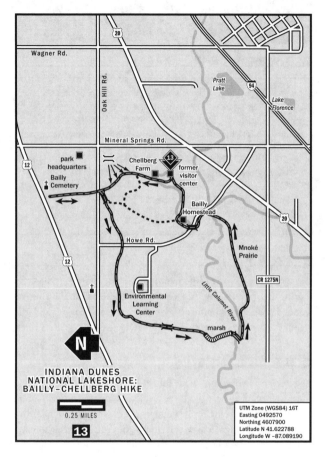

Wagner Rd.

Oak Hill Rd.

20

Pratt Lake

94

Lake Florence

Mineral Springs Rd.

12

park headquarters

Bailly Cemetery

Chellberg Farm

13

former visitor center

Bailly Homestead

20

Howe Rd.

12

Mnoké Prairie

CR 1275N

Environmental Learning Center

Little Calumet River

marsh

N

INDIANA DUNES NATIONAL LAKESHORE: BAILLY–CHELLBERG HIKE

0.25 MILES

13

UTM Zone (WGS84) 16T
Easting 0492570
Northing 4607900
Latitude N 41.622788
Longitude W –87.089190

community in northwest Indiana. Over the years, three generations of Chellbergs made their living on the farm growing wheat, oats, corn, and rye and keeping farm animals. The Chellbergs farmed the land until 1972, when the National Park Service bought the property. To preserve the past, the park service continues operating this typical northwest Indiana farm in the same manner that the Chellbergs operated it in the late 1800s.

The hike starts 100 yards south of the farm, at the backside of the former visitor center, where you'll follow the trail to the right as it runs along the top of a 40-foot wooded ravine. (Unfortunately, in recent years, the visitor center has been shut down.) The first farm building you'll pass is the maple-sugar house, followed by a windmill with a pump house, a harness shop, a corncrib, a chicken house, the restored brick farmhouse built in 1885, and the large 100-year-old barn. Kids will enjoy the roaming chickens, the horses in the barn, and the hogs in the pen beyond the barn. Inside the farmhouse, visitors can tour the parlor, the kitchen, and a bedroom as they looked in the early days of the farm.

Continuing on the trail, cross a bridge and then follow a set of steps down into a pleasant wooded ravine carved by a running stream. Crossing several more bridges, the trail runs along the bottom of the ravine for a short stretch until a flight of stairs brings you back up to flat ground. Cross another bridge and then turn right at the junction for the out-and-back trail to the Bailly Cemetery. On the way to the cemetery, cross Oak Hill Road and a crushed-gravel trail, and then hike 0.3 miles through bottomland forest. The cemetery—a walled-in earthen area built on a small hilltop—has a tomb-like quality to it. The wall was built in 1885 on what archeologists have surmised to be an existing cemetery: bones thought to predate European settlement have been uncovered at this site. After circling the cemetery, retrace your steps back to the main trail.

Back on the main trail, cross a bridge and then stay to the right at the next junction. Soon the trail crosses Howe Road and a crushed-gravel trail that leads to the Indiana Dunes Environmental Learning Center—a frequent stop for school groups visiting the dunes. After passing a spur trail on the left leading to the learning center, you'll see the building on the left through stands of hickory, maple, and locust trees. After passing between a few big white oaks on both sides of the trail, the trail turns left toward the Little Calumet River. From here, the woodland becomes shrubby savanna as the trail runs through a few small ravines.

At 1.9 miles into the hike, a 0.2-mile boardwalk carries you through a wet bottomland forest and a marshland and ends at a scenic spot where a metal footbridge spans the Little Calumet. Stay to the left at a junction 0.2 miles beyond the bridge. After the trail curves left, you'll have sporadic views of the river, marshy areas, and the cattails at the bottom of the ravine. In the riverside areas, ground-cover plants are scarce due to the dense, leafy canopy above. Soon, the trail leaves the riparian landscape behind and enters the 120-acre Mnoké Prairie. After passing through this picturesque prairie and a short stretch of woodland, the trail arrives at a parking area. From the parking area, descend the hill and then stay to the left, heading toward the bridge on Howe Road.

On the other side of the bridge, immediately turn right on the brick road that heads up the short hill to the Bailly Homestead. Montreal-born Honoré Gratien Joseph Bailly de Messein was one of the first settlers in northwest Indiana when he arrived in 1822 to start a trading post. Well suited for trading due to the river and the intersection of two major Indian trails, Bailly exchanged blankets, guns, and cooking pots for skins of beaver, muskrat, and mink. As animals became scarce and the trading slowed, Bailly turned his attention to operating a local tavern and establishing a small community named after him, which was on land now occupied by Bethlehem Steel.

On the right is the restored wooden frame house built by the Bailly family in 1835. Though Bailly died before construction of the house was finished, his family occupied the house until 1917. Over the years, the six-bedroom house has been a restaurant, an antiques shop, and a retreat for an order of Catholic nuns. The ground floor of the house—unfurnished except for a beautiful fireplace mantel built by a local craftsperson—is open to the public on Sundays during the summer. Also on the property are a two-story cabin that served as employee's quarters, a small brick house, a chapel, and a reconstructed fur-trading cabin.

Beyond the house and the cabins, the path on the left, which leads to the Bailly Cemetery, is said to be part of an old Indian trail. The hike continues on the right, just beyond the wigwam frame and the National Historic Marker plaque. From the Bailly Homestead, it's a short woodland hike back to the parking lot.

■ TO THE TRAILHEAD

From Chicago, take I-90/I-94 south until you reach the Chicago
Skyway (I-90), Exit 59A. After traveling 29 miles southeast on the
Skyway and the toll road, take Exit 21 to I-94. Follow I-94 east
for 7 miles until you reach Exit 22B. Follow US 20 (Melton Road)
for 4.1 miles. The entrance to the parking lot is on the left.

 ## 14 *LaSalle Fish and Wildlife Area Loop*

■ OVERVIEW

LENGTH: 5.2 miles

CONFIGURATION: Loop

DIFFICULTY: Moderate

SCENERY: Kankakee River, expansive
marshland, large lake, prairie, savanna,
woodland, and a stream

EXPOSURE: Mostly exposed

SURFACE: Sand-and-dirt two-track road

HIKING TIME: 3–3.5 hours

ACCESS: Much of the west half of this
hike is closed for waterfowl hunting
from October 1 to December 1. If
you're visiting during that time, stick

to the east half of the fish-and-
wildlife area.

FACILITIES: Boat launch at
parking area

MAPS: Map posted at park office;
USGS topos straddle the state
line between Illiana Heights, IL, and
Schneider, IN

SPECIAL COMMENTS: Because this
wildlife area is largely undeveloped,
you're likely to be all alone once you
get away from the prime fishing spots.
Call (219) 992-3019 for more info.

■ SNAPSHOT

If you like riverside hikes and sprawling marshlands, you'll find
them in abundance on this hike, one of the great undiscovered
hikes in Chicagoland.

■ UP CLOSE

About 150 years ago, the Grand Kankakee Marsh was the largest
wetland in the Midwest, stretching for nearly a million acres

through northwest Indiana. Then in the mid-1800s, the marshes were drained, and the Kankakee River was deepened and channelized in order to use the flat, moist landscape for farming. Drainage tiles were installed, ditches were dug, and pumps were installed to push water away from the cropland. Also, an extensive levee system was built to reduce flooding near the waterways. According to the United States Geological Survey, only 13 percent of the Kankakee Marsh remains.

Grand Kankakee Marsh was named by the early French explorers who came through major waterways of the area looking for a water route to the Pacific Ocean. One of these explorers was Robert Cavalier, Sieur de La Salle, for whom the 3,797-acre fish-and-wildlife area is named. LaSalle Fish and Wildlife Area—one of the few original remnants of the Grand Kankakee Marsh—was first established as a state park in the 1960s.

Start the hike in Parking Lot 3A, situated at the edge of a vast, open water marsh called the Black Oak Bayou. Facing the Kankakee River, take the gravel two-track road to the left as it runs along the levee. The levee—which is about 15 feet above the surrounding landscape—provides a bird's-eye view of the river on the right and the marshes and woodland to the left. At 0.2 miles, a large, swampy pond covered with algae and speckled with dead trees opens on the left. Many of these riverside ponds are shaped like short, wriggling worms—indicating their former life as the curves or perhaps the oxbows of the Kankakee before it was channelized. After a brief stretch of cottonwoods and oaks growing in a wet savanna on the left, you'll encounter more marshland alive with swallows soaring among the dead trees, turtles plopping off logs into the water, and lily pads tilting in the breeze.

Once you've logged nearly a mile of hiking, the trail turns left and passes over a bridge spanning a waterway between the marshes on each side of the trail. As the small open marsh on the right turns into an algae-covered ditch and the marsh on the left fades into stands of cattails and willows, the trail turns left again. Prairie grass and compass plants fringe the trail, while willows and cottonwoods hang over the algae-covered drainage ditches

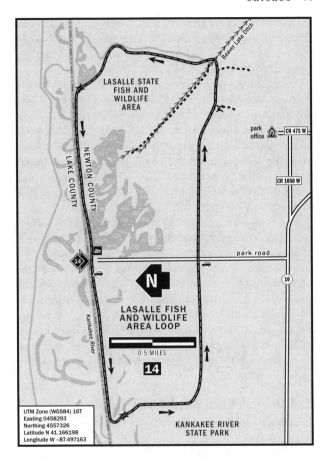

LASALLE STATE FISH AND WILDLIFE AREA

Beaver Lake Ditch

park office

CR 475 W

CR 1050 W

LAKE COUNTY

NEWTON COUNTY

14

park road

10

N

LASALLE FISH AND WILDLIFE AREA LOOP

0.5 MILES

14

Kankakee River

KANKAKEE RIVER STATE PARK

UTM Zone (WGS84) 16T
Easting 0458293
Northing 4557326
Latitude N 41.166198
Longitude W –87.497163

on each side of the two-track road. Beyond the footbridge on the right that provides a connection to Parking Lot 4B, you'll see some cropland peeking through the trees on the left as the trail enters a savanna.

After crossing the road at 2.25 miles into the hike, you'll pass a wet, shrubby prairie with a backdrop of oak woodland on the left. At the point where two-track roads come from both sides, continue straight ahead as the trail angles slightly to the right. Soon, two successive footbridges cross the continuous ditch on the right. Stay on the two-track road as you cross a gravel road and then swing left.

As the trail curves left, Beaver Lake Ditch splits to the right and left, running under the road. Continuing ahead, the trail accompanies a pleasant stretch of the sandy-bottomed creek that gently meanders through wet savanna and woodland. The damp, shady sides of the trail are thick with horsetail grass, the stems of which come apart at their black-fringed joints. After passing a marshy area through the trees on the left, Beaver Lake Ditch flows into the Snag Bayou, which is bordered by quaking aspen and oak. Once you cross a bridge, the trail hits the Kankakee River.

Turning left, finish off the hike with a mile-long stroll between the straight, fast-moving Kankakee River and the immense bayou with stands of dead trees jutting upward and patches of green algae on the surface. Above the cattails and sedge grasses, listen for the loud chattering of belted kingfishers, and watch for them hovering over water as they scout out a meal. The view of the marsh is obscured now and then with berry bushes, small trees, and full-size cottonwoods. In places where the bayou meets the edge of the trail, you'll see that the water level in the marsh is several feet higher that the water level in the river. Continue ahead on the levee until you reach the parking lot.

■ TO THE TRAILHEAD

From Chicago, take I-90/I-94 south. Stay on I-94 as I-90 splits off. When I-94 reaches I-80, continue straight ahead on IL 394 for 4.8 miles. Turn left (east) on US 30 (East Lincoln Highway) and proceed 6.1 miles to US 41 (Wicker Avenue). Hang a right (south) on US 41 and continue 23.8 miles until you reach IL 10 (County Road 1000). Turn right (west) on IL 10 and proceed 2.4 miles until you see the sign for Parking Lot 3A.

OVERVIEW

LENGTH: 2.5 miles

CONFIGURATION: 2 connected loops

SCENERY: Ravines, bottomland, forest, pine plantations, creeks, pond

EXPOSURE: Nearly all shaded

SURFACE: Dirt and some gravel

HIKING TIME: 1 hour

ACCESS: Trails are open 8 a.m.–8 p.m.

FACILITIES: Restroom, water, picnic tables

MAPS: Map signs appear at all trail junctions; paper maps are available in the nature preserve and online at www.fpdwc.org; USGS topo Steger, IL

SPECIAL COMMENTS: Nature center hours are noon–4 p.m., Thursday–Sunday. For more information, call the nature center at (708) 747-6320. A bird checklist is available for free at the nature center.

SNAPSHOT

This lightly used nature preserve is a gem: after exploring the ravines, the pine plantations, the wooded hills, and the streams surrounded by bottomland forest, be sure to check out the former country church that now serves as a nature center.

UP CLOSE

Considering how much it has been hauled around the neighborhood, the little wooden country church that serves as the Thorn Creek Nature Center is in surprisingly good condition. An Emmanuel Evangelical Lutheran congregation built the church in 1862 several miles northwest of its present location. After 100 years, Emmanuel Lutheran gave the church to Village Bible Church of Park Forest, which moved it just north of the nature center off Monee Road. Ten years later, when the Village Bible Church built a new structure, the congregation passed the old church to the Village of Park Forest. The village spruced it up and put it on a new foundation in its present spot.

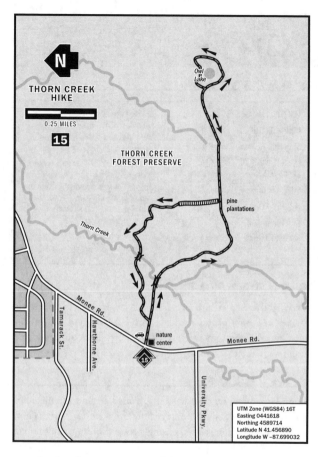

Inside, where generations of churchgoers came to hear ministers' sermons, schoolkids now sit in the pews while park naturalists explain the features of the Thorn Creek Preserve and surrounding areas. The large pulpit, elevated 8 feet above the pews, now contains an action-packed taxidermy scene of a red fox chasing a Canada goose through a cattail marsh. Visitors of all ages will enjoy viewing the nature center's displays of preserved animal specimens;

lichens found in the area; bones, skulls, and arrowheads; photos of animals and plants found in the preserve; and a small nature library in the gallery upstairs. There are also photographs of the farm that occupied the preserve in the early 1900s.

Currently under ownership by the state, the county, and two nearby villages, the nature preserve was formed in the 1960s when private and governmental organizations joined forces to save the property from development.

The hike starts in the backyard of the nature center, on a gravelly path that immediately crosses a bridge over an intermittent stream. As the trail starts to descend a slight hill, watch for the logs half-buried on the trail surface that serve to direct runoff away from the trail. Stay right at the first junction, and you'll soon enter a bottomland forest of black walnut, swamp white oak, basswood, ash, and slippery elm. After passing a second junction on the left, the trail mounts a bridge over Thorn Creek—which may dry up into a series of isolated pools during the summer. Following a short boardwalk, the trail flattens out and winds through a grove of maples.

Soon a shallow ravine develops on the left, and a much deeper 50-foot ravine plunges down on the right. Dominated by maple, ash, and red oak, this ravine contains a tributary of Thorn Creek. As you proceed, listen for wind whispering through groves of red and jack pines planted by farmers in the 1950s (both red and jack pines' needles are in clusters of two, but the red's needles are up to 6 inches long, while the jack's are only 1.5 inches long). According to the bird checklist available at the nature center, these pine plantations provide some of the best birding spots in the 880-acre preserve.

As the path curves left, the landscape flattens and the woods are unwrapped from the dense canopy. In these upland areas, you'll see white and red oak, shagbark hickory, and—after passing the junction with the boardwalk on the left—white pine (needles in clusters of five). On this straight and flat route to Owl Lake you'll see a small cattail pond, pasture roses, and open fields beyond the trees on the right.

After circling Owl Lake (you'll see it's more of a pond than a lake), head back to the junction where the boardwalk starts on the right. While traversing the 0.2-mile boardwalk, you may notice a variety of fern species growing in the wet soil on the sides of the platform. Leaving the boardwalk behind, you'll head back toward Thorn Creek and notice that the landscape begins to drop down on the left. After passing an enormous section of a concrete drain duct, the trail takes a sharp left, drops down the slope, crosses a bridge, and then enters a bottomland forest along a 50-foot section of boardwalk. For the remainder of the hike, look for thick trunks belonging to 150-year-old white and red oaks: the white oaks tend to grow in flat spots, while the reds often grow on the slopes. Stay right at the next two junctions to return to the parking lot.

■ MORE FUN

Just a few miles northeast of Thorn Creek in Cook County is the Sauk Trail Forest Preserve, which includes a 4.7-mile paved path for hiking and biking. The hilly path runs through mature woods, next to ravines, and along the shore of Sauk Trail Lake. From the nature center, head north (turn right) on Monee Road and proceed 1.7 miles. Take a left on South Western Avenue and then quickly turn right on West Sauk Trail. A forest-preserve entrance that accesses the paved path is 0.8 miles ahead on the left.

■ TO THE TRAILHEAD

From Chicago, take I-90/I-94 south. Stay on I-94 until you reach I-57. Follow I-57 south for 18.5 miles to Exit 339. Turn right (east) on West Sauk Trail and proceed 0.9 miles. Turn right (south) on South Cicero Avenue and go 1.9 miles until you reach University Parkway. Turn left (east) and proceed 1.65 miles until you reach Monee Road. Turn left (north) again, and the nature preserve is 0.5 miles ahead on the right.

Public transportation: The University Park station on the Electric Metra Line is located 1.5 miles from the start of this hike. From the station, head east on University Parkway. At Monee Road, turn left. The Thorn Creek Nature Center is just ahead on the right.

■ OVERVIEW

LENGTH: 3.3 miles	4:30 p.m. on weekdays; 10 a.m.– 4:30 p.m. on weekends.
CONFIGURATION: Loop	**FACILITIES:** Nature center, restrooms, picnic tables, and shelters
SCENERY: Bottomland forest, ravines, streams, river, a historic well, and an impressive public greenhouse	**MAPS:** Ask for a trail map at the nature center; USGS topo Joliet, IL
EXPOSURE: Mostly shaded	**SPECIAL COMMENTS:** Contact the nature center at (815) 741-7277. To find out about special flower shows at the Bird Haven Greenhouse, call (815) 741-7278.
SURFACE: Dirt with sections of new pavement and deteriorating asphalt	
HIKING TIME: 1.5 hours	
ACCESS: The park is open dawn–dusk. The nature center is open 9 a.m.–	

■ SNAPSHOT

Pilcher Park offers an appealing mix of graceful ravines, lush bottomland forest, and small winding streams. Toward the end of the hike, you'll see a couple of area landmarks from the 1920s: a still-used public water well and the recently renovated Bird Haven Greenhouse.

■ UP CLOSE

Harlow Higginbotham, an important figure in Chicago during the late 19th century, once owned Pilcher Park. Higginbotham was the president of Chicago's successful Columbian Exposition in 1893, a world's fair commemorating the 400th anniversary of Columbus's arrival in the Americas. After the exposition, Higginbotham used many of the trees that were part of the exhibits to establish a private arboretum on this property. Specimens such as southern magnolia, sweet gum, cypress, tulip tree, pecan, black birch, and various

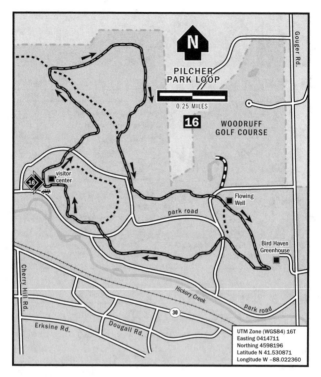

hickories were added to a park that already contained about 75 native species of trees.

In 1920, Higginbotham sold the arboretum to Robert Pilcher, a businessman, self-taught naturalist, and "sturdy pioneer," according to the inscription on his statue near the park's nature center. Eventually, Pilcher donated his 327 acres of virgin woodland to the City of Joliet, with the stipulation that the land be left wild. Higginbotham's name is preserved across the street from Pilcher Park in another park called Higginbotham Woods (see More Fun section).

Thanks to the efforts of Higginbotham and Pilcher, visitors can still explore the park's 420 acres of ravines, streams, and forested bottomland. The ravines roll through the northern section of the park, and the bottomland forest—where you'll see trees such as the bur oak, American elm, and slippery elm—occupies the southern section along Hickory Creek. Come springtime, the landscape in many sections of the park is carpeted with wildflowers.

Your first stop at Pilcher Park ought to be the attractive log cabin–style nature center that hosts a large colorful totem pole, built in 1912, in front. Inside, kids will enjoy the turtle pond; several aquariums containing catfish, sturgeon, crappie, and perch; live snakes; and a live Eastern owl. Also inside is a large window where you can watch the park's birds (and squirrels) feeding at a cluster of bird feeders.

To begin the hike, follow the sign for the North Pilcher Trail on the left side of the parking lot as you're facing the nature center. After the trail dips down to meet the edge of a small pond, follow the sign to the right and then bear left over the footbridge. Just ahead, the trail passes over several drainage culverts before crossing a gravel path and then the park road. On the other side of the park road, the landscape starts to rise.

Reaching the hilltop, the terrain levels out, and the trail curves left and runs above a pleasant wooded ravine containing an intermittent stream. Keep straight ahead at the sign pointing left for the North Pilcher Trail. At 0.6 miles into the hike, where several asphalt trails come together, follow the sign for the Upper Loop Trail on the right. Right away, the Upper Loop Trail enters a flat and dense woodland with a few intermittent streams. After passing an open area where a number of small- and medium-sized trees have been cut, the path starts to lose elevation. Just after crossing a stream, you'll see the beginnings of an expansive wooded ravine on the left. Farther ahead is a nicely situated bench where you can pause and take it all in.

From the bench, the trail descends gradually through a mature oak forest, and then curves right and passes a trail junction. When you reach the gate at the park road, keep straight ahead on the park road until you see the HIKING TRAIL, NO HORSES sign on the left, just before the paved trail that crosses a steel bridge. After taking the hiking trail on the left and then crossing the wooden footbridge, you've suddenly entered a flat bottomland forest. Up ahead, beyond the paved service road, the Woodruff Golf Course appears on the left. Taking a right at the fork leads you over a footbridge, across the park road, and into a picnic area with tables, a shelter, an open grassy area, and the Flowing Well, where you'll likely see a few people filling up their water bottles. The park district maintains that the mineral content and the 51-degree temperature of the water have remained constant throughout the life of the well, drilled in 1927 to a depth of 207 feet. If you don't mind the slight taste of iron and other minerals common in well water, take a drink.

From the well, follow the concrete path left of the restrooms for 0.3 miles to the Bird Haven Greenhouse, which hosts indoor plants and flowers, outdoor formal gardens, seasonal flower shows, and a children's garden. The greenhouse—designed by the same architectural firm that designed the Central Park Greenhouse in New York City—was built in 1929 and underwent a major renovation in 2003. Displayed in front of the greenhouse is the original clock face from the Will County Courthouse, built in 1887 in Joliet.

Proceeding with the hike, find the dirt path at the back of the greenhouse just to the left of the paved path. A quarter mile away from the greenhouse, after passing a small pond and a marshy area thick with shrubs on the left, the trail crosses a park road and a footbridge and then heads back into the bottomland forest. This section of the trail is one of the places in the park where you may see wildflowers such as jack-in-the-pulpit, spring beauty, mayapple, and red trillium. Crossing the park road again, keep straight ahead, soon reaching a footbridge over a small rocky stream. After crossing another footbridge, the trail runs next to the park road and Hickory Creek. At the next trail junction, bear left, and the nature center should be visible through the trees. Cross one final footbridge and then turn left on the interpretive trail that runs toward the backside of the nature center.

■ TO THE TRAILHEAD

From Chicago take I-90/I-94 south. Continue on I-94 until you reach I-57. Take I-57 south for 13.5 miles to I-80 west. After 13.7 miles on

I-80, take Exit 137 and follow US 30 (West Lincoln Highway) for 0.6 miles left (west). Turn right (north) on South Gouger Road and follow it for 0.3 miles until you see the first of two entrances for the park on the left. Take either entrance and follow the signs pointing toward the nature center.

Public transportation: Pilcher Park is 2.5 miles from the New Lenox station on the Rock Island Metra line. From the station, head north on North Cedar Road. Turn left on West Francis Road. West Francis Road ends at the Bird Haven Greenhouse.

■ MORE FUN

Higginbotham Woods, also owned by the Joliet Park District, is across Gouger Road from Pilcher Park. You can walk an old gravel road that traverses the park from east to west. This is accessible from Francis Road, which heads west from Gouger Road just south of the Bird Haven Greenhouse. Near the parking area is a large boulder with an inscription describing a French fort that was allegedly built on this land in 1730 and a trading post built in 1829. Recent archeological studies show, however, that the supposed indications of an early French fort are actually irregularly shaped earthworks created by Native Americans of the Hopewell period, which ranges from 200 BC to AD 400.

■ OVERVIEW

LENGTH: 2.4 miles

CONFIGURATION: Loop

SCENERY: Tallgrass prairie, marshes, ponds, historic cabin, observation deck

EXPOSURE: Completely exposed

SURFACE: Mowed grass

HIKING TIME: 1.25 hours

ACCESS: The park is open from sunrise to sunset; the visitor center is open 10 a.m.–4 p.m.

FACILITIES: Restrooms, picnic areas, a beverage vending machine, and a visitor center with exhibits

MAPS: Park map usually available outside visitor center; USGS topo Coal City, IL

SPECIAL COMMENTS: Pets must be leashed. Contact the visitor center at (815) 942-2899 or visit www.dnr .state.il.us.

■ SNAPSHOT

While making your way through this hypnotic tallgrass prairie, you'll skirt the edges of several marshes and ponds active with birds. For those interested in improving their prairie plant–identification skills, this hike offers a nice variety of grasses and flowers, as well as some interpretive signs to get you started. Near the end of the hike, the trail passes a reconstructed version of one of the earliest log homes in the county.

■ UP CLOSE

There's a good reason that Illinois is the nation's top producer of soybeans and the second largest producer of corn—it's the sea of grass that once dominated the state. It wasn't just any grass that made the soil so fertile, but big, hearty tallgrasses like big bluestem, Indian grass, and prairie cordgrass. Thousands of years of these grasses rotting on the ground created rich, dark soil more fertile than other grasslands farther west. Along with being more fertile, tallgrass prairies are considered by many to be the most dramatic type of grassland. This is especially true during mid- to late summer, when

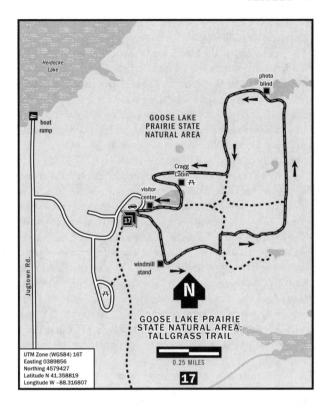

UTM Zone (WGS84) 16T
Easting 0389856
Northing 4579427
Latitude N 41.358819
Longitude W –88.316807

GOOSE LAKE PRAIRIE STATE NATURAL AREA: TALLGRASS TRAIL

0.25 MILES

17

10-foot-high grasses and an abundance of flowers decorate these vast spaces.

Unfortunately, Illinois's agricultural dominance has come at a cost. With only 0.5 percent of the state's surface area remaining as tallgrass prairie, it seems the "Prairie State" nickname is now a misnomer.

One of the best places to experience the dramatic beauty of these big open grasslands and gain a better understanding of how they function is within the Chicago region. As the largest tract of tallgrass prairie in the state, Goose Lake Prairie State Natural Area gives visitors a taste of what it looked like when grassland covered two-thirds of the Illinois.

Before starting the hike behind the visitor center, take in the view from the observation platform attached to the back of the building. If it's July, the prairie will be exploding with wildflowers of all shades; if it's September, goldenrod and compass plants will form a yellow carpet over the landscape. A few miles to the northeast, you'll see the Dresden Nuclear Power Plant (as you're hiking, you'll also notice another power plant, the Midwest Collins Generating Station, a couple miles to the west).

From the map board at the bottom of the platform's ramp, take the mowed trail on the right winding through the prairie. In the wet areas you'll see Indian grass, prairie cordgrass, and sedge grasses. Big bluestem grass—perhaps the most common of tallgrass prairie plants—lines the trail. Sometimes called "turkey foot" for the arrangement of its seed heads, big bluestem grows most attractively in the late summer, when it reaches heights up to 10 feet and takes on various colors, from steely gray to wine red to muted lavender. In earlier times, livestock happily munched on big bluestem within this prairie. At 0.2 miles into the hike, you'll see evidence of the grazing that once took place here in the old windmill stand that pumped water out of the ground for the livestock.

After you pass a couple of smaller, cattail-fringed marshes— one with open water—a sign indicates that the trail heading to the right is closed. You can still proceed ahead but must turn back once you reach the marsh, because a bridge is in need of repair. Taking the next right brings you to the other side of the marsh, where a rebuilt covered wagon with a bench inside is situated on a slight rise above the open water. Given the scarcity of trees near the pond, the wagon's canopy provides a welcome shady spot when the sun is hot overhead. In the vicinity of this marsh, I've seen great blue herons, a kingfisher, and a foot-long snapping turtle that became utterly peeved when I attempted to touch its shell.

From the pond, stay to the right as you start the large rectangular loop. During the summer, tall compass plants grow on this section of trail, as do small crab apple trees and an attractive grass called Canada wild rye, which has a large, bushy, nodding seed head. Also, black-willow shrubs grow near the patches of open water on the left side of the trail. As the path curves left, a cattail marsh with open water appears on the right. The enclosed photo blind provides benches and small viewing doors that allow you to discreetly observe action in the marsh. After passing another marsh on the right, look for obedient plants (lavender, tubular flowers lined up on the stalk) during late summer. This northern section of the park is dominated by Indian grass, which is often hard to identify until August, when the reddish-brown tassels and small yellow stamens come into bloom.

Finish the rectangular loop by turning right on the gravel trail, which leads along the backside of the Cragg Cabin, a replica of one of the first homes in Grundy County. The next left takes you to the cabin. Originally built by the Cragg family in 1830 and located south of the park along the Mazon River, the cabin became a stopover for travelers and for cowboys who herded cattle from St. Louis to the stockyards of Chicago. The cabin, which sits at the edge of this pleasant pond bordered by a quaking aspen and willows, has been reconstructed a couple of times, most recently in 1980 by the Youth Conservation Corps. The small interior of the cabin is laid out much as it would have been 175 years ago, with a bed frame, a fireplace, and a ladder leading up to a second-floor loft. Stay to the right after the cabin, and you'll hike along the edge of the pond back to the visitor center.

■ TO THE TRAILHEAD

From Chicago, take I-90/I-94 south to I-55. Follow I-55 south for 51 miles until you reach Exit 240. Take Pine Bluff–Lorenzo Road to the right (west) for 2.9 miles. Turn right (north) at the sign for Goose Lake Prairie State Natural Area (North Jugtown Road). Proceed ahead for 1 mile and then turn right (east) at the sign for the visitor center.

■ MORE FUN

Interested in more prairie hiking? If so, there is a 2.8-mile hike that runs south from the Goose Lake Prairie visitor-center parking lot.

At the south end of the hike, you'll climb on top of a mound left over from a former coal-mining operation in the park.

Not far from Goose Lake Prairie, the town of Morris hosts Gebhard Woods State Park, a small but pleasant park that adjoins a stretch of the Illinois and Michigan Canal Trail. Inside the park, the 0.8-mile Nettle Creek Nature Trail runs along the winding creek and through stands of maple, cottonwoods, and sycamores. On the east side of the park, toward downtown Morris, is an old stone aqueduct where the I&M Canal flows over Nettle Creek. Morris, the seat of Grundy County, situated on the north bank of the Illinois River, was one of many towns that grew up alongside the I&M Canal. To reach Gebhard Woods from Goose Lake Prairie, take Pine Bluff Road to the right (west) for 5 miles to IL 47. Turn right (north) on IL 47, continuing over the river and into Morris, and turn left (west) on County Road 2 (West Jefferson Street). Proceed 0.9 miles and turn left (south) on Ottawa Street. The park is just ahead on the left.

18   Matthiessen State Park Dells Area Hike

■ OVERVIEW

LENGTH: 2.2 miles	**FACILITIES:** Picnic tables, pavilion, water, flush toilets
CONFIGURATION: Loop with out-and-back segment	**MAPS:** Park maps are available at trailhead; USGS topo LaSalle, IL
SCENERY: Sandstone canyons, waterfalls, wooded bluffs, lake, high footbridges over creek	**SPECIAL COMMENTS:** Cross-country-ski rentals are available December–March when weather permits. Maps at horse-trailer parking areas show the routes for 13 miles of equestrian trails available at Matthiessen. Horse rentals are available on IL 71, a half mile west of IL 178.
EXPOSURE: All shaded	
SURFACE: Gravel, dirt	
HIKING TIME: 1.5–2 hours	
ACCESS: 8 a.m.–sunset	

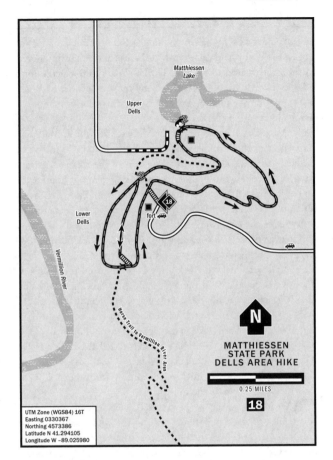

MATTHIESSEN STATE PARK DELLS AREA HIKE

0.25 MILES

18

UTM Zone (WGS84) 16T
Easting 0330367
Northing 4573386
Latitude N 41.294105
Longitude W –89.025980

■ SNAPSHOT

Formerly a private retreat for a local industrialist, Matthiessen State Park features a narrow, mile-long canyon carved in sandstone by a stream. Beginning at the dam and lake at one end of the canyon, you'll encounter a couple of dramatic waterfalls while exploring the moist and shady canyon floor and the wooded bluffs above.

■ UP CLOSE

Overshadowed by the far-more-popular Starved Rock State Park 2 miles to the north, Matthiessen State Park is often unjustly ignored by the many visitors to the area. The latter park's 1,938 acres don't offer as many miles of trails or as many canyons as Starved Rock, but they still have plenty of geological charm—not to mention a much quieter atmosphere.

A LaSalle businessman named Frederick William Matthiessen, who reportedly employed some 50 people to build the trails, bridges, stairways, and dams, first developed the area as a private park. Matthiessen also built a not-so-modest summer home with 16 bedrooms and 9 baths, along with a smaller mansion for one of his children. While Matthiessen's structures no longer remain, visitors will see the handiwork of his grounds crew in the dams, stairs, and soaring concrete footbridges. By 1940, 22 years after Matthiessen's death, his heirs donated the property to the state.

Similar to Starved Rock's, the beautiful sandstone walls at Matthiessen were carved out by centuries of flowing water. The mile-long canyon at Matthiessen is nearly 100 feet deep in places and ranges from 50 to 140 feet wide. The section closest to the dam and Matthiessen Lake is called the Upper Dells, and the path of the canyon closest to the Vermilion River is called the Lower Dells. (The canyons here were called dells during Matthiessen's time— since then the name has stuck.) A dazzling 40-foot waterfall separates the two sections of the canyon.

From the parking lot, head toward the small log fort, which is a replica of forts the French built in the Midwest during the 1600s and early 1700s (the French constructed one of these forts on Starved Rock in 1683). Start the hike by heading down the stairs and taking the first trail to the right. This wide, elm-lined gravel trail follows the bluff above the creek deep within the sandstone canyon on the left. At 0.2 miles, as the path starts to curve, you'll begin to see rock on the other side of the canyon and hear a couple of waterfalls down below. Stay to the left as you pass over the creek, which flows through a culvert under the trail (the trail to the right leads to the horse-trailer parking area).

Continuing on the other side of the canyon underneath a canopy of sugar-maple trees, the trail soon becomes paved. Before crossing the bridge over Lake Falls, pay a visit to the overlook on the left for your first view of the Lake Falls as it drops 40 feet from the top of a dam to the floor of the canyon. After crossing the bridge, which provides a nice view of the wooded banks of Matthiessen Lake and the falls underneath, the first trail on the left brings you down closer to the falls and then descends to the floor of the Upper Dells.

On the canyon floor, you can gingerly step through a mix of sandstone, rock, and mud to get a better view of the falls. Mosses, liverworts, and ferns grow on the damp, shady, 30- to 40-foot walls of the canyon. Farther along in the canyon, solid sandstone channels the stream over a small waterfall that empties into the pool called the Giant's Bathtub. Geologists say these pools develop and grow larger by the action of rocks and pebbles getting swirled around. As you continue ahead, several places require using boards and rocks to cross the stream. As the canyon curves to the right at a place called Cedar Point, continue ahead past stairs leading up to the bluff.

Farther ahead, take the stairs out of the canyon and then follow the sign for the Lower Dells and proceed along the bluff, passing Cascade Falls on the left. After walking along the bluff, cross the bridge and follow the stairs to the Lower Dells. The short box canyon on the right is called the Devil's Paint Box, because the walls are decorated with swaths of yellow, orange, and brown, formed by minerals seeping out of sandstone. In the main canyon, look for spots where lichen has changed the rock to light green. Look for changes in the texture of the walls, too: some sections are smooth and flat, while others are rough, pitted, and almost grotesque. The cracks in the walls form much like the cracks in pavement during the winter, growing bigger and chipping apart when water freezes inside.

As on the Upper Dells, the trail here alternates between mud and rock and requires stream crossing via large rocks and concrete blocks. More trees grow in this canyon, particularly sugar maples, some of which are draped with vines. At the end of the canyon, listen for the soothing echo created by the 40-foot waterfall. Frederick Matthiessen named his private retreat Deer Park in honor of the

Native American practice of using these canyons for confining deer. Heading back up the stairs, turn left at the sign for the fort and parking lot. Turning right at this junction leads to the Vermilion River Area within the park (see More Fun section). Heading toward the parking lot, the trail rises and then curves left. Complete the hike by climbing the stairs back up to the parking lot.

■ TO THE TRAILHEAD

From Chicago, take I-55 to I-80. After driving 45 miles on I-80, take Exit 81 south to Utica. Proceed south along IL 178 for 5.1 miles, passing through Utica and over the Illinois River. The entrance to the Dells Area at Matthiessen State Park is on the right, just south of IL 178.

■ MORE FUN

South of the Dells Area, the Vermilion River Area within the park offers 1.9 miles of hiking along the wooded bluffs above the river. While there are no canyons in this section of the park, there is exposed rock in places, and there is a striking view from a high bluff. Visitors can drive to the Vermilion River Area by heading south on IL 178 from the Dells Area entrance. A better way to make the trip, if you have the time and energy, is to take the mile-long horse trail, which starts on the right after emerging from the Lower Dells.

For more canyon hiking, head over to Starved Rock State Park, located 2 miles north. From the Starved Rock visitor center, some shorter trails will take you up on platforms offering expansive views of the Illinois River. Because Starved Rock is the busiest state park in Illinois, consider visiting early in the day or during the week—the trails often get congested at peak times.

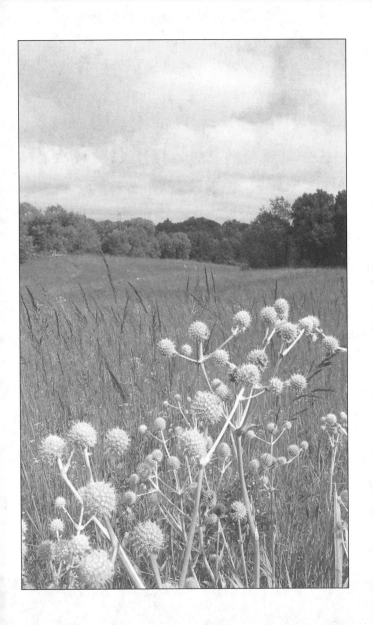

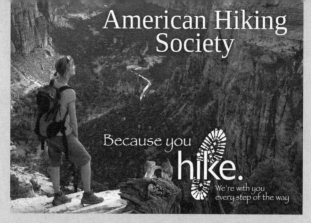

American Hiking Society

Because you hike.
We're with you every step of the way

Since its founding in 1976, **American Hiking Society** has been the only national voice for hikers—dedicated to promoting and protecting America's hiking trails, their surrounding natural areas and the hiking experience. **American Hiking Society** works every day: Speaking for hikers in the halls of Congress and with federal land managers; Building and maintaining hiking trails; Educating and supporting hikers by providing information and resources; Supporting hiking and trail organizations nationwide.

Whether you're a casual hiker or a seasoned backpacker, become a member of **American Hiking Society** and join the national hiking community! You'll not only enjoy great members-only benefits but you will help ensure the hiking trails you love will remain protected and will be waiting for you the next time you lace up your boots and hit the trail.

We invite you to join us today!

American Hiking Society

1422 Fenwick Lane · Silver Spring, MD 20910 · (800) 972-8608
www.AmericanHiking.org · info@AmericanHiking.org